Best Minnesota
Camper Cabins

Roughing It in Comfort

Tom Watson

Adventure Publications
Cambridge, Minnesota

ACKNOWLEDGMENTS

First and foremost, I want to thank all the staff throughout the Minnesota DNR's State Park system for their cooperation during this project. Special thanks to Erik Wrede, my friend and "go-to" source, who always puts me in contact with the right people, no matter what. One of those special people is Peter Hark, Operations Manager for the DNR who helped set up contacts and provided me with snippets of info throughout the process. Thanks, too, to all the agency people at other units who provide camper cabins: National Forests, county and regional parks, and a few private vendors as well. I also want to thank my lifelong friend and traveling buddy, Craig Swedberg, who joined me on many outings throughout the state as head navigator. Sharing these jaunts from cabin to cabin with a dear friend who appreciates our parks as much as I do is the most fulfilling aspect of these projects. Special thanks to my sister, Lynn, for providing me with a base to work out of whenever I am doing field research in or near the Twin Cities. She's been there for every guidebook project.

Lastly, I want to thank you, the reader, and hope you find the camper cabin opportunity to be yet one more way to enjoy all that our incredible park system—and great state— have to offer.

Edited by Brett Ortler

Cover and book design by Lora Westberg

Photo credits
All photos courtesy of Tom Watson or via Shutterstock unless otherwise noted. All photos copyright of their respective photographers.

Front cover: "Sandy Beach" cabin by Tom Watson **Back cover:** Chippewa County Park (top right inset), Savanna Portage State Park (bottom photo) by Tom Watson; Jay Cooke State Park (bottom inset) by Minnesota DNR

Anne Arthur: 11 (top three), 15 (top), 24 (top), 25, 27 (bottom), 30 (bottom), 51 (bottom) **Joshua Borchardt:** 123 (bottom) **Camp Tanadoona/Camp Fire Minnesota:** 141 (both) **Michelle Kohlgraf:** 21 (bottom), 24 (bottom), 30 (top), 58, 93 (top), 99 (bottom), 118, 120 (top), 136

The photos on the following pages are copyright by the Minnesota Department of Natural Resources and used with permission; DNR photographers are specified if known: 10, **Erik Pelto**; 11 (bottom), **Kristen Anthony**, 23; 71, 72 (top), 73, 98, **Erik Pelto**, 132, 135; 139 (bottom three)

10 9 8 7 6 5 4 3 2 1

Copyright 2017 by Tom Watson
Published by Adventure Publications
An imprint of AdventureKEEN
820 Cleveland Street South
Cambridge, Minnesota 55008
(800) 678-7006
www.adventurepublications.net
Printed in U.S.A.
ISBN: 978-1-59193-721-0; eISBN: 978-1-59193-722-7

PREFACE

There's something about a cabin in the woods. Maybe it's images of Thoreau at Walden Pond or Sigurd Olson writing from his Listening Point cabin on Lake Burntside. Whatever the inspiration, a cabin is the quintessential retreat in the woods—safe, secure, cozy, and quiet—all in a setting of rustic, northern beauty.

Minnesota may be the "Land of 10,000 Lakes," but it probably has thousands of cabins as well, and at times it seems like everyone's "going up to the cabin for the weekend." Of course, not every cabin is created alike: Some of these cabins are fully furnished with all the luxuries of home, some look like motels or hotels perched along the edge of a northern lake, and a few are well off the beaten track.

And then there are "camper" cabins. Essentially serving as a place to sleep, get out of the rain, and avoid the bugs, these simply furnished structures are a notch up from camping in a tent, but they still stay in touch with the outdoor camping experience.

For the seasoned outdoor enthusiast they offer a cushy upgrade from hard-core tent camping; for the beginner, they provide a chance to test your camping mettle in stages, allowing you to hone your camping skills at your own pace, while always having a roof and a bed to retreat to when needed.

We all have our own sense of what a cabin means to us, and these places provide more than 100 different ways to experience that feeling throughout Minnesota.

Table of Contents

INTRODUCTION

Using Minnesota's state park cabins as a model, a "camper" cabin is a unit that offers bare facilities: a set of bunk beds and a table and chairs or benches; some may have electricity and/or heat (even woodstoves in some cases), but that's it! There's no plumbing. You can plug in a coffeemaker or slow cooker, but there are no other appliances or setups for kitchens, and indoor cooking is usually not allowed. (The one exception is at the National Forest cabins at East Bearskin Lake on the Gunflint Trail, where you are allowed to use a cookstove in the cabin.)

There are more than 100 cabin units that meet those criteria. They are found throughout Minnesota. Many are located in state parks, but several are found in county or regional parks, and a few are even run by private vendors. And while these cabins share many of the same types and styles of furnishings, each has its own setting and personality, and that's really what puts them in a class of their own.

I've ranked the camper cabins in this book; I judge each cabin on how private, scenic, quiet, and secure it is. When it comes to how private and quiet a cabin is, I take its proximity to other cabins, campers, and high-traffic areas (roads, popular trails) into consideration. I judge a cabin's setting and security based on where the cabin is situated in a given park; some are within campground loops, some are adjacent to campgrounds, and still others are in separate sections of the park, out of earshot and out of view of other campers.

Each cabin account includes details about where you can access fresh water (both seasonally and year-round), as well as where the nearest outhouses, restrooms, and shower facilities are. I also list a few amenities that the cabins offer. as well as a general description of the attractions in the park and surrounding area. Also included are the rates and reservation process, as well as contact information for the park unit.

GPS coordinates are furnished for either the park entrance or the entrance to the cabins —or in some cases, both. All these cabin sites are well marked; find the park and you'll find signage directing you to the cabins.

Finally, each listing offers my notes on the individual cabins or other pertinent information about these units. "Tom's Tip" suggests a particular activity or attraction that is especially noteworthy about the park or area in which these cabins are located.

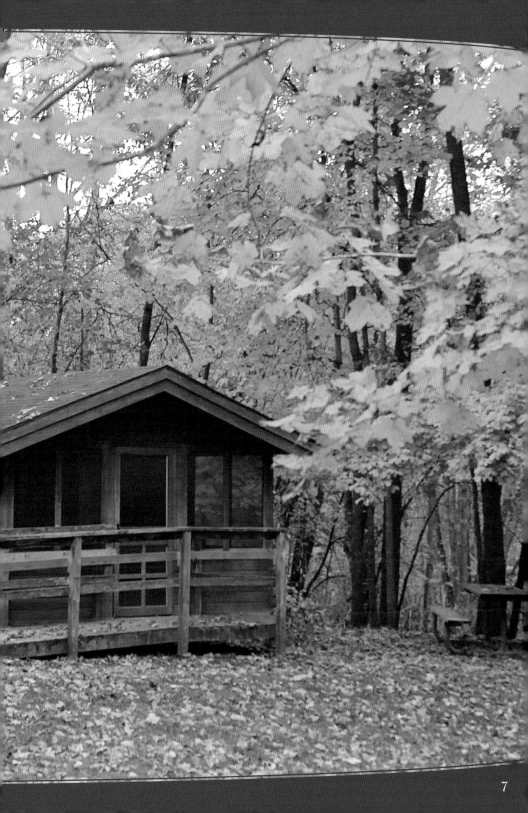

Fees and Deposits

Renting a camper cabin is relatively inexpensive, and cabin rates vary slightly depending on the amenities they offer and when you're staying. At the cabins in Minnesota's State Park system, you can expect to pay the following amounts/night.

Basic cabins (no electricity): Sun.–Thurs. $55/night; Fri.–Sat. $65/night

Cabins with electricity (electricity and/or heat): Sun.–Thurs. $60/night; Fri.–Sat. $70/night

Making Reservations

Reserving a Minnesota State Parks Cabin is as easy as a phone call or going online. Reservations can be made 24 hours a day, except for the first day a reservation becomes available. On that first day, reservations cannot be made online before 8 a.m.

A nonrefundable reservation fee ($10 for call center/$8.50 for web) is charged for each advance reservation. There is no reservation fee to reserve a same-day campsite. The reservation fee (if applicable) and camping fees for the entire length of stay must be paid when the reservation is made.

Phone Reservations

To reserve by phone, call 866-857-2757; TTY: 218-336-2189.

The call center is open the following hours:

April-September: Daily, 8 a.m.–8 p.m.

October-March: Mon.–Fri., 8 a.m.–6 p.m.; Sat.–Sun., 8 a.m.–2 p.m.

The call center is closed on holidays.

Online Reservations

Making reservations online is a snap. You can check availability by location and make a reservation in minutes. To do so, you'll need to create an account. To get started, visit https://reservations1.usedirect.com/MinnesotaWebHome/

If you need to cancel or modify your reservation, you can do so online or by contacting the call center. Modifications will incur a charge ($5 online/$7 via the call center). You can also cancel your stay; if you cancel four days or more prior to your arrival, you'll be charged a cancellation fee of $10. If you cancel less than four days prior to arrival, you forfeit the first night's camping fee and will be charged a $10 cancellation fee. (You'll be refunded the rest of the deposit, except for the nonrefundable reservation fee.)

Also, if a campsite is not occupied on the first night of a reservation, the reservation will be canceled. The first two nights' camping fees are forfeited and a $10 cancellation fee is charged. The customer is refunded the remaining amount of the deposit minus the nonrefundable reservation fee.

Check-in, Check-out and Pets

- Check-out tiime is at 1 p.m.
- Check-in time is at 3 p.m.
- Pets are not allowed in camper cabins

What To Bring

Overnighting in a camper cabin is just like camping out in a tent. You will need all the same gear, but with perhaps a few extras. Here's a list of suggested items to help make your cabin experience even more enjoyable.

- **Slow cooker and coffee maker** Except for warming up or creating meals in a slow cooker and brewing coffee, all cooking must be done outside the structure (including screened or covered porches). Fire rings and picnic tables are provided at all cabin sites.

- **Small table; camp chairs** All cabins are furnished with table/chair/bench units, but having a spare table and a few extra chairs will be handy too.

- **Bed coverings/linens** Cabins all have comfortable mattresses (twin and double) but no linens. Sleeping bags, pillows, and/or conventional bed coverings are best options.

- **Slippers, casual footwear** Most all cabins have warm wooden floors, so having comfortable footwear around the cabin is a cozy option to consider.

- **Games, entertainment** Board games, decks of cards and other forms of table-top activity are ideal for those cabin-bound days/evenings.

- **Housekeeping gear** Many cabins do have brooms, dust pans, etc., but it's your responsibility to tidy up the cabin during your stay and upon your departure.

- **Electronics.** Cabins with electricity have outlets; otherwise, bring spare batteries. Cabin walls let you crank up the volume a bit more, but remember, you may have cabin neighbors close by.

- **Miscellaneous.** Any gear that you always wanted to bring camping but didn't want to keep in the tent.

Camper Cabin Destinations, By Interest

The camper cabins in Minnesota's State Parks are as varied as the parks themselves. Some are situated amid birding or angling hotspots, whereas others are perfect for those seeking out some privacy and a nice secluded spot to rest. If you've got a specific pursuit or a type of stay in mind, check out the following lists!

Best for Biking

- Afton State Park
- Bunker Hills Regional Park
- Lake Bemidji State Park
- True North Basecamp Cabins

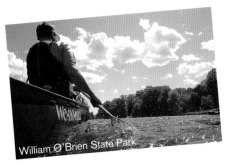
William O'Brien State Park

Best for Canoeing/Kayaking

- Banning State Park
- Bear Head Lake State Park
- Chippewa County Park
- Crow Wing State Park
- East Bearskin Lake National Forest Campground
- Glendalough State Park
- Hayes Lake State Park
- Maplewood State Park
- Myre-Big Island State Park
- Savanna Portage State Park
- Wild River State Park
- William O'Brien State Park

Best for Fishing

- Beaver Creek Valley State Park
- Big Bog State Recreation Area
- Chippewa County Park
- Glendalough State Park
- Maplewood State Park
- Mille Lacs Kathio State Park
- Savanna Portage State Park
- Whitewater State Park

Best for Groups

- Forestville State Park
- Glacial Lakes State Park
- Lake Bemidji State Park
- Lake Carlos State Park
- True North Basecamp Cabins
- Sibley State Park

Best for Hiking

- Afton State Park
- Banning State Park
- Elm Creek Park Reserve
- Jay Cooke State Park
- Lake Maria State Park
- Savanna Portage State Park
- William O'Brien State Park
- Wild River State Park

Best for Kids
- Bunker Hills Regional Park
- Flandrau State Park
- Hok-Si-La Municipal Park
- Lake Koronis County Park

Best for Privacy/Seclusion
- Elm Creek Park Reserve
- Glendalough State Park yurt
- Hayes Lake State Park
- Lake Maria State Park
- Maplewood State Park
- Tall Pines yurt
- "Sandy Beach" Cabin

Best for Swimming
- Bunker Hills Regional Park
- Flandrau State Park

Best for Unique Attractions
- Banning State Park
- Big Bog State Recreation Area
- Bunker Hill Regional Park
- Flandrau State Park
- Forestville State Park/Mystery Cave
- Jay Cooke State Park
- Minneopa State Park
- Sibley State Park

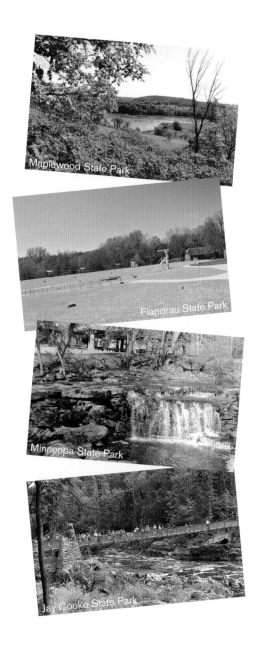

Maplewood State Park

Flandrau State Park

Minneopa State Park

Jay Cooke State Park

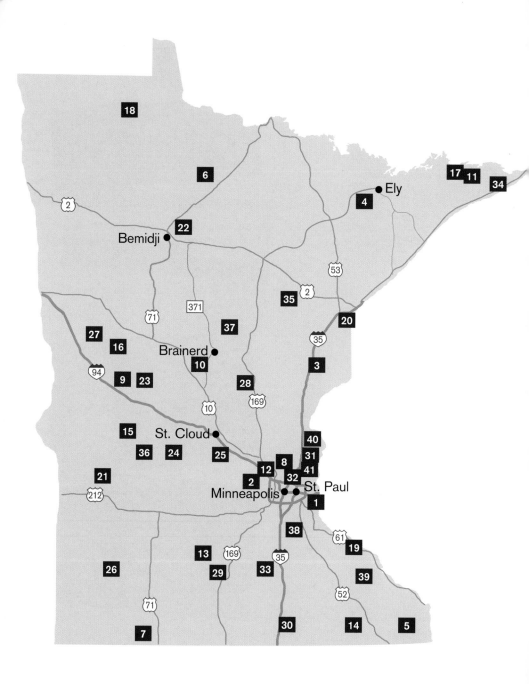

18

6

Ely

17 11

34

2

4

22

Bemidji

35

2

53

20

371

37

35

71

27

16

Brainerd

3

10

94

9 23

28

169

10

15

St. Cloud

40

36 24

25

31

41

12 8

32

2

Minneapolis

St. Paul

21

1

212

38

61

19

13

169

39

26

29

33

35

52

71

30

14

5

7

1. Afton State Park
2. Baker Park Reserve
3. Banning State Park
4. Bear Head Lake State Park
5. Beaver Creek Valley State Park
6. Big Bog State Recreation Area
7. Brown Park South
8. Bunker Hills Regional Park
9. Chippewa County Park
10. Crow Wing State Park
11. East Bearskin Lake National Forest Campground
12. Elm Creek Park Reserve
13. Flandrau State Park
14. Forestville State Park/Mystery Cave
15. Glacial Lakes State Park
16. Glendalough State Park
17. Gunflint Pines Cabins
18. Hayes Lake State Park
19. Hok-Si-La Municipal Park
20. Jay Cooke State Park
21. Lac Qui Parle State Park
22. Lake Bemidji State Park
23. Lake Carlos State Park
24. Lake Koronis County Park
25. Lake Maria State Park
26. Lake Shetek State Park
27. Maplewood State Park
28. Mille Lacs Kathio State Park
29. Minneopa State Park
30. Myre-Big Island State Park
31. Ojiketa Regional Park
32. Rice Creek Chain of Lakes Park Reserve
33. Sakatah State Park
34. "Sandy Beach" Cabin
35. Savanna Portage State Park
36. Sibley State Park
37. True North Basecamp Cabins
38. Whitetail Woods Regional Park
39. Whitewater State Park
40. Wild River State Park
41. William O'Brien State Park

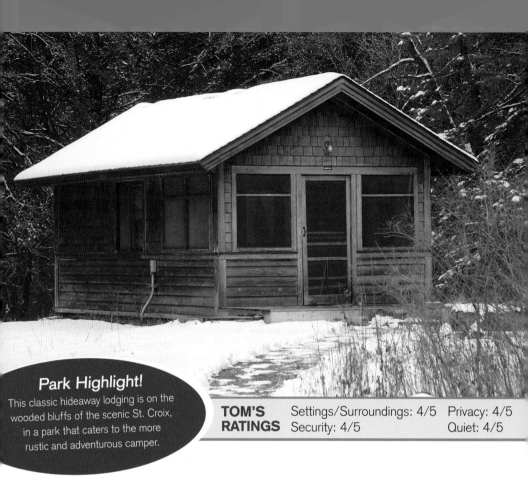

| **TOM'S RATINGS** | Settings/Surroundings: 4/5 | Privacy: 4/5 |
| | Security: 4/5 | Quiet: 4/5 |

Number of cabins/availability: 4 cabins, 2 yurts; available year-round.

Cabin sleeping capacity: **Cabins:** *Big Bluestem* and *Bur Oak* sleep 6; *Bluebird* and *White Pine* sleep 5 and are ADA accessible; **Yurts:** *Gray Fox* and *Coyote* sleep 7 (both ADA accessible).

Cabin features: **Cabins:** Electricity, heat, table/benches, bunk beds, a light strip over each bunk, fire ring, and picnic table; **Yurts:** No electricity. Heat via a woodstove (firewood provided), table/chairs, rocking chair, bunk beds, fire ring, picnic table, and a food preparation shelter.

Where to find water/bathrooms: **Cabins:** There is a vault toilet between *Big Bluestem* and *Bluebird* cabins; seasonal water is found by the *Bur Oak* parking area; year-round water is available across the road at the parking area for yurts. **Yurts:** A vault toilet and year-round water are adjacent to the parking lot at the walk-in entrance to yurts.

Water and flush toilets are available at the Visitor Center year-round, but there are no shower facilities in the park.

Reservations/fees: 866-857-2757; www.dnr.state.mn.us
  Cabins: Sun.–Thurs. $60/night; Fri.–Sat. $70/night
  Yurts: Sun.–Thurs. $60/night; Fri.–Sat. $65/night

Restrictions: No cooking, pets, or smoking.

GPS: Entrance to park, 44.847837,-92.797605; entrance to cabins/yurts area, 44.844421,-92.775898

Key information: Afton State Park, 6959 Peller Avenue South, Hastings, MN 55033, 651-436-5391, www.dnr.state.mn.us/state_parks/afton/index.html

Area activities/attractions:

With more than 20 miles of hiking trails and 4 miles of bike trails, all accessible via trailheads near the cabins/yurts, this park is perfect for hikers and bikers. The trails make their way along bluffs and along the banks of the St. Croix River, a state-designated Wild and Scenic River.

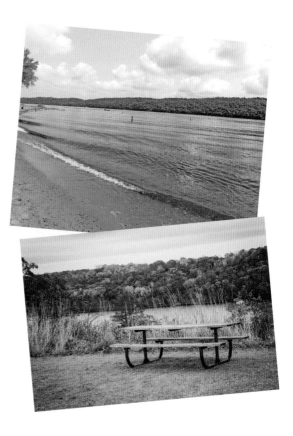

Nearby Afton Alps ski area offers mountain bike courses in addition to its slopes during winter. In winter, the Visitor Center rents out snowshoes. Afton Alps Golf Course is also part of the cluster of outdoor attractions neighboring Afton State Park. Retail shopping in the town of Afton is just 10 miles away too.

Notes: Afton State Park epitomizes low-impact camping, or for that matter, low-impact outdoor recreation in general: the amenities and features in this park are accessible only by foot, bike, or canoe/kayak.

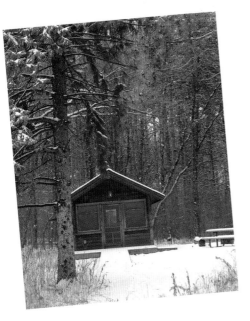

The cabins, yurts, and group camp clustered in the southeast section of the park are the only camping options accessible by car. To reach the park's campground, you've got to backpack in!

Each cabin is tucked under a thick canopy of pines, spruce, and an occasional oak just beyond the group campground parking area. They all enjoy a limited view out past the road and across the grasslands, where you'll see the park's two yurts in a clearing. Together, the cabins and yurts offer remote, rustic lodging reminiscent of frontier settlements in Minnesota's north country.

Afton State Park is a hiker's park, offering more than 20 miles of trails that weave, loop, and cross through a network of pathways. The trails boast a wide variety of scenery: Some dip and bend through the wooded bluffs or wind through open fields 300 feet above the river, while others head across prairie-like grasslands in the north section of the park or the pine plantations in the southern end. Better yet, a full 2 miles of trails follow the western shoreline of the St. Croix. All in all, it's a challenging trail system, making hiking or snowshoeing a great way to enjoy the park.

TOM'S TIPS: This park offers both highland terrain and meandering pathways through the river lowlands and along the banks of the St. Croix River, offering a lot of variety. As cabins are adjacent to the Afton Alps Ski Area, they are a great place for skiers to stay in winter, and the same is true for mountain bikers who race down Afton's slopes during the summer. Both should find these cabins a restful retreat after a day of attacking the slopes in any season.

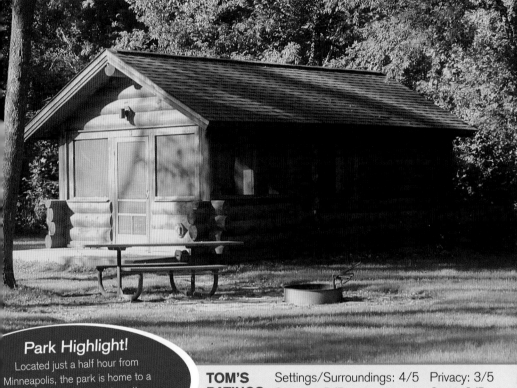

Park Highlight!
Located just a half hour from Minneapolis, the park is home to a row of cabins situated along the treelined edge of a well-groomed campground.

TOM'S RATINGS

Settings/Surroundings: 4/5   Privacy: 3/5
Security: 5/5   Quiet: 3/5

Number of cabins/availability: 5; seasonal (Apr.–Oct.).

Cabin sleeping capacity: Cabins 1 and 2 sleep 5 (ADA accessible); Cabins 3–5 sleep 6.

Cabin features: Electricity, heat, overhead lighting, ceiling fans and outlets, bunk beds, fire ring, picnic table, screened porch, and ample parking.

Where to find water/bathrooms: Restrooms, showers, and a dishwashing station are available in the adjacent campground (Loop A); water is available where Loops A and B intersect with the park road, and at the park office near the entrance.

Reservations/fees: Required. Call 763-559-6700. $60/night.

Restrictions: No cooking, pets, or smoking.

GPS: Entrance to cabin loop in Campground A, 45.0182878, -93.637302

Key information: Baker Park Reserve, 2309 Baker Park Road, Maple Plain, MN 55359, 763-694-7860, www.threeriversparks.org/parks/baker-park.aspx

Area activities/attractions: Visitors can enjoy a wide range of summer activities, including archery, biking, boating, fishing, geocaching, hiking, swimming, golf, or enjoying a relaxing lunch at the park's picnic area.

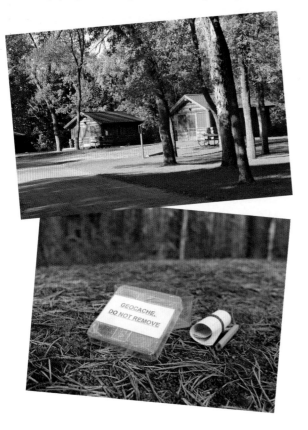

Notes: The five cabins at Baker Park Reserve sit on the uppermost loop of an expansive campground near the southeast shore of Lake Independence. The string of cabins is spaciously situated along the campground road loop with their front doors facing out towards the tent/RV campground. Glimpse out the back window, however, and you'll see the woods and a shaded understory provided by a thick stand of oaks, maples, and other hardwoods.

Cabin 1 commands a key position at the edge of the trees right at the north end of the loop and is closest to the campground office, which doubles as a drinking water source and the trailhead for several trails. Cabins 2–4 and 5 enjoy a smattering of shade trees in their front yards.

Baker Park offers a wide variety of recreation options, many of which take place in the large recreation area located along the shore of Lake Independence. Easy to access on the park roads, it's located just north of the cabins.

Just southeast of the cabins is an access trailhead for the paved, 6.2-mile hiking/biking trail around Lake Katrina. It's a fairly level route that showcases the park's woodlands, grasses, and marshy areas.

TOM'S TIPS: The Baker Near-Wilderness Settlement is a unique attraction in the park. Basically a group camp featuring 8 cabins, a lodge, and even a rock wall, it offers a variety of outdoor programs for groups, as well as a few "Camper Cabin Weekends" each season. During these events, families can experience cabin camping and learn about a variety of aspects of this style of camping, or learn outdoor skills like archery, orienteering, and even making fire the old-fashioned way. Wilderness Settlement activities and courses are separate from other Baker Park activities.

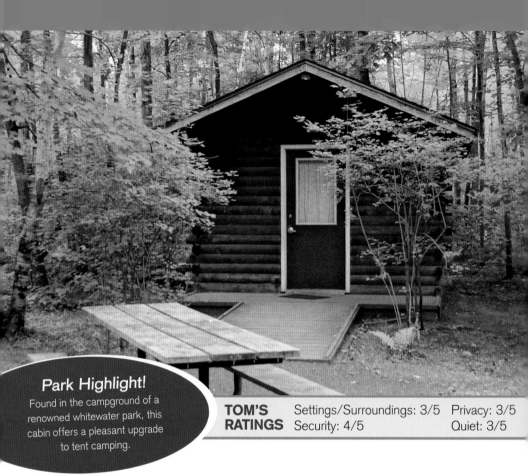

TOM'S RATINGS Settings/Surroundings: 3/5 Privacy: 3/5
Security: 4/5 Quiet: 3/5

Number of cabins/availability: 1; seasonal (Apr.–Oct.).

Cabin sleeping capacity: 5

Cabin features: No electricity or heat; bunk beds, a table and benches, fire ring, and picnic table.

Where to find water/bathrooms: All facilities, including a restroom and showers, are located in the campground loop, just a few campsites away; water is available year-round at the park office.

Reservations/fees: 866-857-2757; www.dnr.state.mn.us; Sun.–Thurs. $55/night; Fri.–Sat. $65/night.

Restrictions: No cooking, pets, or smoking.

GPS: Park entrance, 46.179692, -92.848754

Key information: Banning State Park, P.O. Box 643, Sandstone, MN 55072, 320-245-2668, www.dnr.state.mn.us/state_parks/banning/index.html

Area activities/attractions: The park is famous for its natural amenities, including a series of falls and rapids, and it's also home to 14 miles of hiking trails, 11 miles of skiing trails, and 5 miles of snowmobile trails.

Notes: Situated amid the park's two campground loops, this cabin has the same spaciousness that the surrounding tent sites enjoy. The area's thick understory and plants help give each site privacy, and the longer driveway to the cabin keeps road traffic at a comfortable distance.

The cabin is a simple structure and lacks a porch, but it has a roomy clearing out front for the table and fire ring. Adjacent campsites might be in hearing range, but they are clearly out of sight from this cozy cabin. Located right in the campground loop, the cabin is a comfy upgrade to a night in a tent.

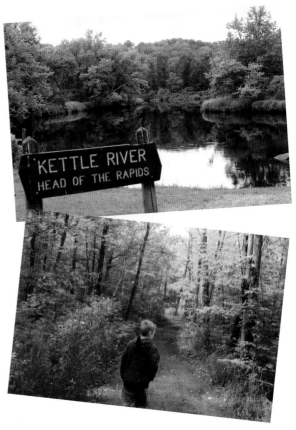

The key feature of this park is the Kettle River, with its roaring rapids, cascades, and raging currents, all of which make the park a paradise for experienced whitewater paddlers. The Kettle River flows along the park's entire eastern boundary and features a landscape dotted with exposed rocks, with some cut sharply by the course of the river. Other sections offer more tranquil stretches of water.

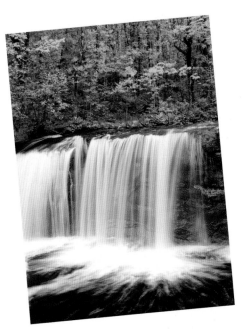

If you're not a river rat, hiking along the shore or fishing in the Kettle River are great ways to enjoy the park. If you plan to spend time on the river, one highlight of the whitewater is the Banning Rapids and Hell's Gate, a raging, narrow passage where the Kettle River has cut through 40 feet of solid bedrock.

TOM'S TIPS: Even non-paddlers still can enjoy the thrill of these rapids and the surrounding scenery by taking the trails that head out from the campground and following the river upstream and downstream. A 10-mile stretch of the Kettle River flows through the park, and trails follow most of its course. The park is also home to a historic sandstone quarry site near Hell's Gate; it provided sandstone to buildings all over the state, and a town—Banning—sprang up next to it. Sandstone soon fell out of favor, and Banning became a ghost town.

Bear Head Lake State Park

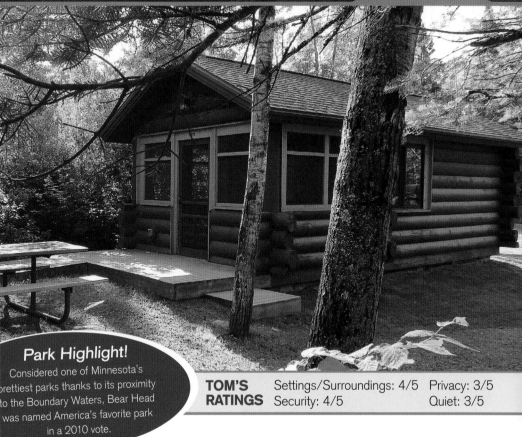

Park Highlight!

Considered one of Minnesota's prettiest parks thanks to its proximity to the Boundary Waters, Bear Head was named America's favorite park in a 2010 vote.

TOM'S RATINGS

Settings/Surroundings: 4/5 Privacy: 3/5
Security: 4/5 Quiet: 3/5

Number of cabins/availability: 5; year-round.

Cabin sleeping capacity: *Red Pine* and *White Pine* sleep 6; *Aspen*, *Cedar*, and *Birch* sleep 5.

Cabin features: Electricity, heat, table/benches, fire ring, picnic table, and screened porch.

Where to find water/bathrooms: Water and a vault toilet are available in the cabin loop between *Red Pine* and *Birch* cabins. Water is available in the campground (mid-May–Sept.); year-round water is available at the park office and in the Trail Center. Vault toilets are accessible year-round in the campground, and flush toilets are available in the Trail Center year-round. Showers are available mid-May through Sept. and are located just a short distance across the road from *Cedar* cabin.

Reservations/fees: 866-857-2757; www.dnr.state.mn.us; Sun.–Thurs. $60/night; Fri.–Sat. $70/night.

Restrictions: No cooking, pets, or smoking.

GPS: Park entrance, 48.189623, -92.047779; Entrance to cabin loop, 47.792768, -92.083858

Key information: Bear Head Lake State Park, 9301 Bear Head Lake State Park Road, Ely, MN 55731, 218-235-2524, www.dnr.state.mn.us/state_parks/bear_head_lake/index.html

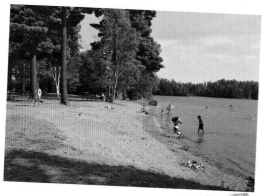

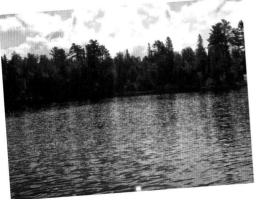

Area activities/attractions: The park also has dock facilities; boat, canoe, and kayak rentals; numerous wilderness trails (including access to Taconite State Trail) as well as remote campsites accessible only via the water. Supplies and services are just 15 miles away in Ely.

Notes: These five cabins—*Red Pine, Aspen, Birch,* and *Cedar* on one loop, and *White Pine* just to the west—are situated across from the campground and located on the North Bay of Bear Head Lake. *Red Pine* and *Aspen* cabins are especially well situated as their front porch areas face away from the road; the other three are just off the main park road, but all are located under a forest canopy of pines and mixed northern hardwoods.

All of the cabins are just a few steps away from the water, and there are plenty of ways to enjoy the lake. There's a small beach beyond the campground and docks line the shoreline, providing plenty of access points. The lake itself offers more than 23 pristine miles of shoreline to explore. Because this is a back-country-style park, many trails lead to remote sites at nearby lakes, and it's also a great park for hiking thanks to its Boundary Waters-like environment. And that's not just a selling point: This is one of a few Minnesota parks where you might actually get to see a wolf, and you're more than likely to hear one! It's also an angling destination as its lakes are home to crappies, walleyes, and bass; Cub Lake is even stocked with brook trout!

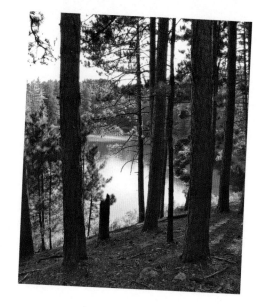

TOM'S TIPS: When you're in the area, consider a visit to the International Wolf Center in Ely. Protecting the Gray Wolf, a true icon of North Country wildlife, the exhibits, programs, and live "wolf ambassadors" on site provide visitors with fascinating insights into this king of the Minnesota forests. Also, after a night in a cabin, consider camping in one of the park's remote backcountry, walk-in, or paddle-in sites.

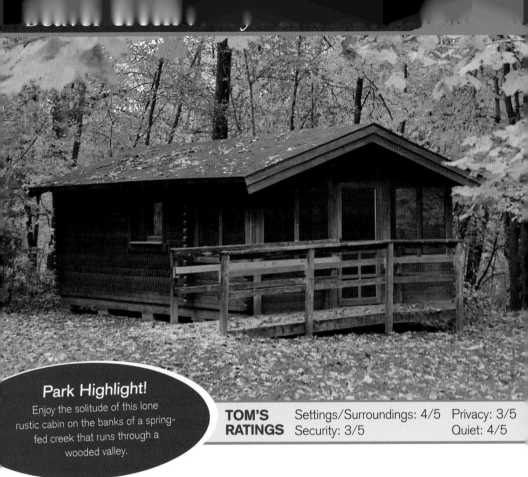

Park Highlight!

Enjoy the solitude of this lone rustic cabin on the banks of a spring-fed creek that runs through a wooded valley.

TOM'S RATINGS
Settings/Surroundings: 4/5　Privacy: 3/5
Security: 3/5　Quiet: 4/5

Number of cabins/availability: 1, seasonal (mid-April–mid-Oct).

Cabin sleeping capacity: 5

Cabin features: Electricity, electric wall heater and fan, table, bunk beds, fire ring, picnic table, access ramp, and screened porch.

Where to find water/bathrooms: The water source is adjacent to cabin; restrooms/showers are nearby, just along the campground road.

Reservations/fees: 866-857-2757; www.dnr.state.mn.us; Sun.–Thurs. $60/night; Fri.–Sat. $70/night.

Restrictions: No cooking, pets, or smoking.

GPS: Park office, 43.644444, -91.578916

Key information: Beaver Creek Valley State Park, 15954 County Road 1, Caledonia, MN 55921-8653, 507-724-2107, www.dnr.state.mn.us/state_parks/beaver_creek_valley/index.html

Area activities/attractions: Camping, 8 miles of hiking trails, wildflowers, trout fishing, birding, and a natural spring all attract visitors.

Notes: What's not to like about a solitary rustic cabin alongside a babbling, spring-fed creek that runs through a virgin hardwood forest? That's what you get at Beaver Creek, which is situated amid the steep slopes of this southeastern Minnesota valley.

This region is part of Minnesota's driftless area—an area unaffected by the glaciers that scoured other parts of the state. Here, in what is known as the Blufflands Landscape Region, you'll find towering valley walls that rise 250 feet above its floor. The hiking trails within the park follow the contours of the valley, meandering alongside the banks of the streams in the park.

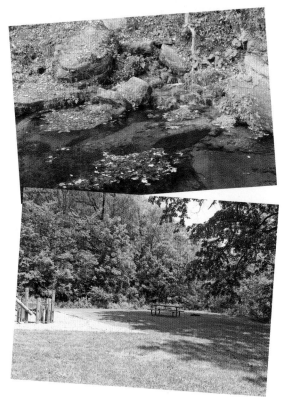

Set back into the lowland forest of black ash, willow, and cottonwood that lines the banks of Beaver Creek, the cabin here faces a large open lawn that blends gracefully towards the treelined creek. A scattering of maple and basswoods create a golden canopy over the cabin in the fall, while in spring the babbling sound of the creek filters through its windows.

A pathway leads from the edge of the cabin clearing to a small pool that formed where crystal-clear spring water flows out of the ground. Fresh watercress grows in this pool year-round. Depending on the season, the creek itself flows intermittently here, but springs also bubble up through the sandstone layers along East Beaver Creek near the campground and picnic shelter building.

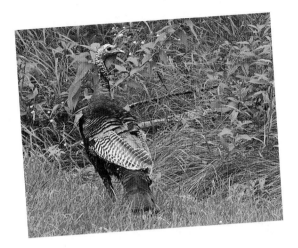

In spring, visitors will find the wooded hillsides flush with wildflowers and birdsong. Songbirds, including the rare Acadian flycatcher, cerulean warbler, and Louisiana waterthrush, migrate into the valley; this is the only place in Minnesota where you're likely to see these species. Valley wildlife includes deer, raccoon, muskrat, mink, badger, red fox, and gray fox. Occasionally beaver and wild turkeys are observed in the park, too.

TOM'S TIPS: Brown and native brook trout inhabit the park's streams, which are considered some of the best trout waters in the state. In fact, this entire southeastern portion of the state is noted for its fine trout streams and paddling.

A NOTE OF CAUTION: Cabin and campground users should be aware of the possibility of flash flooding in the park's creeks after a heavy rain. Park staff will offer specific instructions in the event that an evacuation is necessary. Also be aware that venomous timber rattlesnakes are found in the park, so it's best to always stay on designated trails.

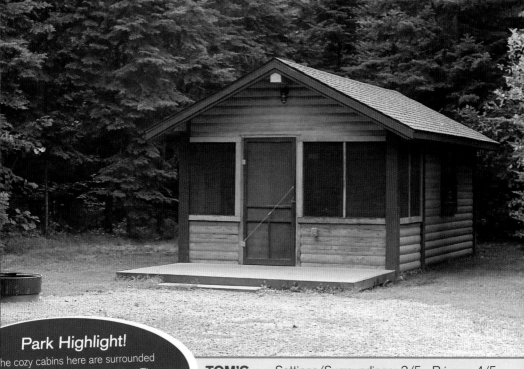

Park Highlight!
The cozy cabins here are surrounded by incredible fishing and neighbor The Big Bog, one of America's greatest natural treasures.

TOM'S RATINGS

Settings/Surroundings: 3/5   Privacy: 4/5
Security: 3/5   Quiet: 4/5

Number of cabins/availability: 5; year-round.

Cabin sleeping capacity: Cabin 1 sleeps 5 (ADA accessible); Cabins 2–5 sleep 6.

Cabin features: Electricity, heat, ceiling fan, table/benches, bunk beds, and screened porch.

Where to find water/bathrooms: Seasonal water is available near Cabin 1, just beyond Cabin 5; water, restrooms, and showers are also available at the nearby campground.

Year-round water is available at the maintenance building; a family-style modern shower and restrooms are located in the Visitor Center.

Reservations/fees: 866-857-2757; www.dnr.state.mn.us; Sun.–Thurs. $60/night; Fri.–Sat. $70/night.

Restrictions: No cooking, pets, or smoking.

GPS: Entrance to park/Southern Unit, 48.170824, -94.512621; entrance to Northern Unit Bog area, 48.286464, -94.553743

Key information: Big Bog State Recreation Area, 55716 Highway 72 NE, Box 428, Waskish, MN 56685, 218-647-8592, www.dnr.state.mn.us/state_parks/big_bog/index.html

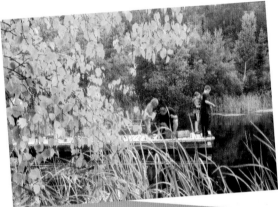

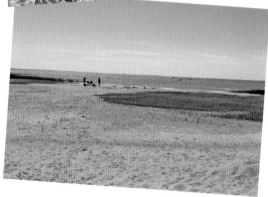

Area activities/attractions: The park is home to two separate units—the Northern Unit and the Southern Unit. At the Southern Unit, visitors enjoy swimming, a sandy beach, fishing in the Tamarac River and Upper Red Lake, camping, canoeing and kayaking (with rentals at the Visitor Center), a boat ramp, a picnic area, a playground area, and a snowmobile trail. There is also a nearby fish hatchery and short hiking trails. A publicly accessible fire tower is located behind the Visitor Center.

The Northern Unit features a mile-long boardwalk through the largest peat bog in the Lower 48 states as well as other hiking trails. It's home to a multitude of plants and myriad wildlife-viewing opportunities.

Notes: Situated amid a smattering of northern pines, spruce, and jack pine, Big Bog's cabins are located in the Southern Unit of the recreation area, and they are laid out in a row between the Tamarac River and the nearby state highway. The huge turnouts in front of the cabins provide ample parking as well as space for the picnic table and the fire ring.

Inside, the buildings seem to glow thanks to the golden knotty pine décor that truly befits a North Woods cabin, and each is furnished much like the cabins you'd find at any other state park. Each cabin is spaced far enough apart to provide a sense of solitude, yet it's just a short walk to the Visitor Center and all the amenities of the campground and river.

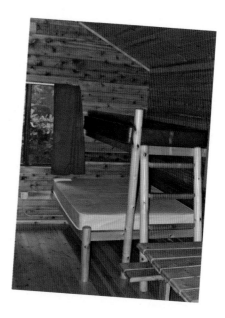

The modern Visitor Center has great interpretive displays about the Northern Unit of the recreation area. The center also features modern, family-style restrooms and showers and serves as a water source year-round. There's also a fire tower on site, which provides a great view of the campground and cabins area and the western expanses of Upper Red Lake and of the Tamarac River to the east.

Nine miles north of the cabins you'll find the 500-square-mile peat bog—the largest of its kind in the Lower 48. A mile-long boardwalk through the heart of this expansive bog brings visitors to within feet of rare plant life, including orchids and even carnivorous plants. More than 300 species of birds have been observed here. In addition, this area is habitat for moose, wolves, bear, and other northern Minnesota mammals.

TOM'S TIPS: The area surrounding the cabins is a popular and highly productive fishing spot, particularly during the spring northern pike season. Boating on the Tamarac River that flows through the recreation area or on massive Red Lake itself are great ways to experience nature.

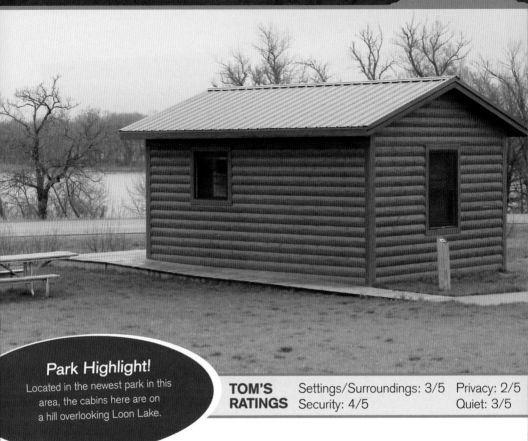

Brown Park South

Park Highlight!
Located in the newest park in this area, the cabins here are on a hill overlooking Loon Lake.

TOM'S RATINGS
Settings/Surroundings: 3/5   Privacy: 2/5
Security: 4/5   Quiet: 3/5

Number of cabins/availability: 4; seasonal (May 1–Oct. 31.) There are also cabins open for special reservations in the fall during hunting season (but no running water is available in the park during that time).

Cabin sleeping capacity: All cabins sleep 5 (1 queen, 3 twin).

Cabin features: No heat; 18' x 15' space, electricity, floor fan, ceiling fan, table/chairs, mini refrigerator, coat hooks, fire ring, and deck.

Where to find water/bathrooms: Restroom facilities are located within the nearby campground loop, and two drinking water faucets are located between cabins.

Reservations/fees: Reservations required. Call 507-847-2525, ext. 7250, or visit www.co.jackson.mn.us and search for the park and fill out the reservation form. One night: $40; weekly: $225; $40 deposit.

Restrictions: No smoking; pets allowed, but no damage allowed from pets; maximum 6 people for sleeping; cabin condition is to be left in same condition as found; no excessive drinking, partying, or roughhousing allowed; follow all other campground rules; no grills on the deck.

GPS: Entrance to campground, 43.524883, -95.107808

Key information: Jackson Co. Parks Department, 53053 780th Street, Jackson, MN 56143, 507-847-2525, ext. 7250 (parks office, cabin reservations, payments, questions), www.co.jackson.mn.us

Area activities/attractions: Park features include a picnic area, a playground, a boat dock, and an asphalt bike-hike trail to nearby Robertson Park, which connects to the 55-mile trail system in Dickinson County.

Notes: Located just over the border from Iowa's popular Lake Okoboji Recreational Area, the cluster of county parks in the lakes region of Jackson County in Minnesota provide many recreational opportunities. One of five county park units in the area, Brown Park South is the only one to feature camper cabins. While each is equipped with a mini refrigerator, the cabins here are otherwise your basic few-frills camper cabins and are furnished with the standard bunk bed and a table and chairs.

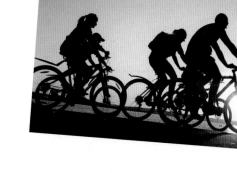

The cabins are perched on a grass-covered hill just across the highway from Loon Lake. Beyond road traffic and sounds drifting over from the campsites, the cabins are otherwise quiet and peaceful with only the other nearby cabins to contend with.

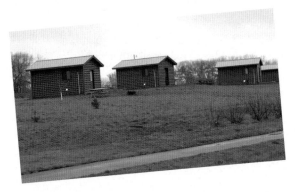

The cabins themselves are well-built, tidy structures in great condition, and they're easy to access, just a short walk from their own dedicated parking area. They're also not far from the restroom and shower facilities within the campground loop. The hub of the park features a playground with picnic tables, and the park's network of bike trails connects with other nearby county parks. All in all, the nearby park system and lake scenery give the place a pleasant country atmosphere that's ideal for families seeking a relaxing evening with a bit more comfort than tent camping.

TOM'S TIPS: Head here if you're a bicyclist. Bringing a bike gives you access to the entire park, and there are dozens of miles of connecting trails. After you spend the day pedaling, the cabins are an appealing overnight option.

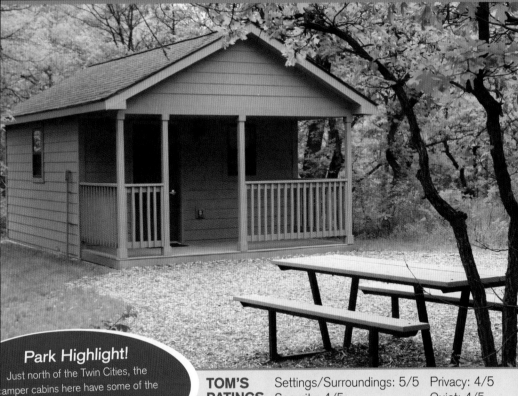

TOM'S RATINGS Settings/Surroundings: 5/5   Privacy: 4/5
Security: 4/5   Quiet: 4/5

Number of cabins/availability: 2; seasonal (Apr.–early Oct.); off-season camping is in effect Oct. 10–23 (no bathrooms/showers/water available, but portable toilets available in campground).

Cabin sleeping capacity: 5

Cabin features: Electricity, baseboard heat, 14' x 16' units with natural pine walls, ceiling fan, ceiling lights, table/benches, log-framed bunks with matresses, lights above each bunk, and a covered porch.

Where to find water/bathrooms: Water is available next to cabin site 38, and a shower and restrooms are a short distance away in the adjacent campground loop.

Reservations/fees: 763-757-3920. A park permit is also required. Daily permits are $5; annual permits are $25 and honored at all Anoka County regional parks as well as regional parks in Washington and Carver counties. $55/night; $8 reservation fee.

Restrictions: Each cabin has a maximum capacity of 6 guests. Visitors younger than 18 must be accompanied by an adult; all vehicles must have a park permit; garbage and recycled materials must be separated and placed in appropriate dumpsters; and there is no smoking, cooking, or pets allowed in cabins. Fires are only permitted in fire pits.

GPS: Cabin location, 45.209209, -93.279614

Key information: Bunker Hills Campground Visitor Center, 13101 County Parkway B, Coon Rapids, MN 55433, 763-862-4970, www.anokacounty.us/910/Camping

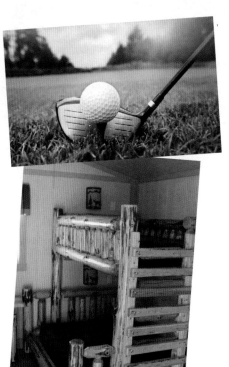

Area activities/attractions: Nearby attractions include an 18-hole golf course, Bunker Beach Waterpark, an archery range, and riding stables. There is also a network of biking and hiking trails throughout the park.

Notes: The classic rustic interiors of these cabins glow thanks to the golden hues of the pine log furnishings. From the bedposts to the table leg and everything in between, these are some of the most beautiful camper cabins in Minnesota, and they are as solid, secure, and comfy as they first appear. The layout is a standard floor plan offering table/benches and two sets of bunk beds. Large lights over each bunk add to the brightness, creating a warm glow reminiscent of a small fireplace.

The cabins are situated among the campsites in the Rustic Loop camping section, a more spacious and woodsy arrangement of sites within the larger campground complex. Located just beyond the outer edge of the suburban ring around the Twin Cities, the oaks and pine-forested hills in this park are the perfect setting for a cabin. Spacious front yards and long and broad driveways create a niche of privacy within the heart of the campgrounds.

There are more than 5 miles of trails winding over the hills and through the forests here. Horse stables provide options for an equestrian experience, and for a more urban thrill, cabin campers and others are drawn to the huge water park just west of the camping area. Add in an archery range and an 18-hole golf

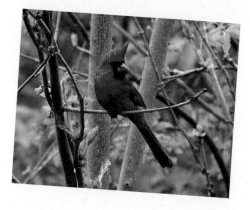

course and you have an incredible amount of options, just minutes away. Don't miss the long boardwalk that heads out over a marsh; it's a great spot for birding.

TOM'S TIPS: Quickly accessible from the Twin Cities, these cabins are a delight to the eye, especially for someone who has memories of quaint, rustic pine-timbered cabins far up north. Majestic stands of oaks intermixed with pines throughout these rolling hills and knolls is the perfect setting for a quick north woodsy escape from the urban buzz just a few miles south.

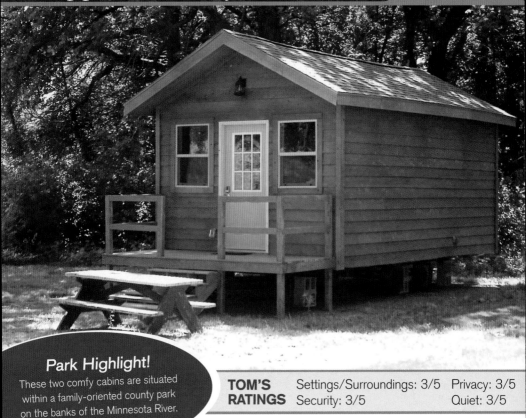

Park Highlight!

These two comfy cabins are situated within a family-oriented county park on the banks of the Minnesota River.

TOM'S RATINGS

Settings/Surroundings: 3/5 Privacy: 3/5
Security: 3/5 Quiet: 3/5

Number of cabins/availability: 2; year-round.

Cabin sleeping capacity: 6

Cabin features: Electricity, heat, small counter space, ceiling fan, table/chairs, bunk beds, sleeper couch, fire ring, picnic table, and small deck.

Where to find water/bathrooms: A vault toilet is located near the cabin, but no water is available at site; it's available in nearby Montevideo.

Reservations/fees: Reserve online at www.lodgix.com/10481/?theme=1; the cabins are labeled as the "Wegdahl cabins" on the website. $50/night.

Restrictions: No cooking or pets in cabin.

GPS: Entrance to park/campground, 44.892268, -95.650311

Key information: Chippewa County, 629 No. Eleventh Street, Montevideo, MN 56265, 320-269-6231.

Area activities/attractions: The park features a playground, a pavilion, a boat launch, campsites, and 6 miles of paved bike trails between park entrance and Montevideo.

The cities of Montevideo (north) and Granite Falls (south) have retail establishments and professional services; nearby Lac Qui Parle and Upper Sioux Agency State Parks offer hiking trails, boating, river fishing, bicycling, and cross-country skiing.

Notes: Spanning 30 acres, Chippewa County Park is located 6 miles south of Montevideo in a grove of bur oaks, maple, and basswood trees along the Minnesota River. The park features a playground, a DNR boat ramp to the river, and two relatively new camper cabins that were modeled after those found in Minnesota's state parks.

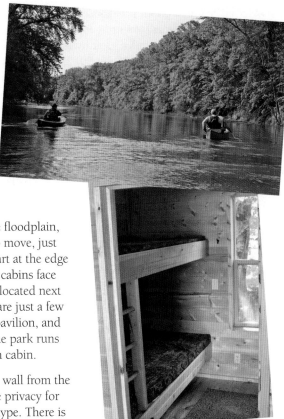

Because the park is situated in the floodplain, the cabins were built to be easy to move, just in case. Sitting about 30 yards apart at the edge of the large, open-space park, the cabins face out towards the main parking lot located next to the playground area, and they are just a few steps away from the picnic area, pavilion, and a group fire ring. A road within the park runs right up to the front porch of each cabin.

The bunk beds are separated by a wall from the main room providing a little more privacy for sleepers than most cabins of this type. There is also a sleeper sofa in the main living area.

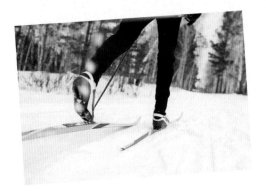

In addition to the paved bike/hike trail between the park and Montevideo, the Bushwackers, a group of Montevideo outdoors enthusiasts, maintain a 3.5-mile cross-country skiing loop beginning in the park. Its trailhead is adjacent to the cabins and extends southward beyond the park's boundaries. This group has been very instrumental in the development of this county park.

TOM'S TIPS: Canoers and kayakers can enjoy a few hours floating one of the river's many scenic corridors by putting in upstream at Prien's Landing (GPS: 44.929726, -95.726753) on Montevideo's southwest side and then taking out at the landing at Chippewa County Park (GPS: 44.891277, -95.650072, which is about 8 miles downstream and has a paved parking lot, a dock, and a wash-down pad (to prevent the spread of invasive species). This entire section of the Minnesota River is teeming with catfish and other fine catches, and fishing from the riverbank is a two-minute walk from the cabins.

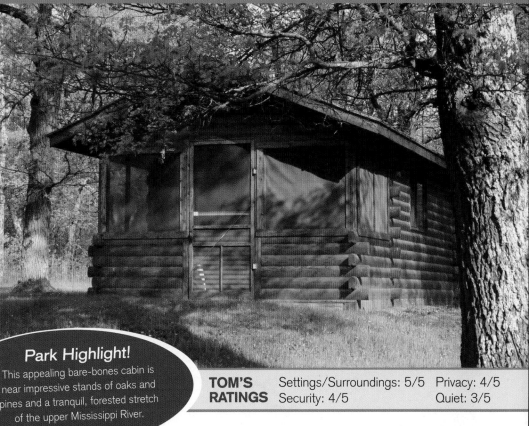

Park Highlight!

This appealing bare-bones cabin is near impressive stands of oaks and pines and a tranquil, forested stretch of the upper Mississippi River.

TOM'S RATINGS

Settings/Surroundings: 5/5   Privacy: 4/5
Security: 4/5   Quiet: 3/5

Number of cabins/availability: 1; seasonal (Apr.–Oct.).

Cabin sleeping capacity: 5 (ADA accessible)

Cabin features: No electricity or heat; table, bench, and bunk beds.

Where to find water/bathrooms: Water is available across the road; the nearest toilets and showers are 100 yards away in the campground loop.

Reservations/fees: 866-857-2757; www.dnr.state.mn.us; Sun.–Thurs. $55/night; Fri.–Sat. $65/night.

Restrictions: No cooking, pets, or smoking.

GPS: Entrance to park, 46.263936, -94.318512; entrace to cabin, 46.279269, -94.328251

Key information: Crow Wing State Park, 3124 State Park Road, Brainerd, MN 56401, 218-825-3075, www.dnr.state.mn.us/state_parks/crow_wing/index.html

Area activities/attractions: There are 14 miles of hiking trails within the park as well as boating and fishing on the Mississippi and Crow Wing Rivers. Several historic sites are found in the park, including Old Crow Wing Village and a section of the famous Red River Oxcart Trails that once crisscrossed the state.

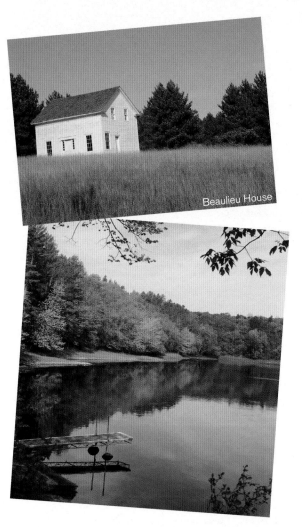

Beaulieu House

Notes: The road into the cabin winds through healthy stands of oaks and red pines, a preview of what to expect when you reach the site. Sitting within a stand of majestic pines, the cabin is found on an open, grass-covered slope just before the entrance to the campgrounds.

It's a most appealing setting: it's spacious, shaded by the towering pines, and with a large open yard. It's also just far enough off the park road to offer a bit of privacy. That being said, you will experience traffic nearby as the cabin is located just before the main loop of the campground.

The screened porch faces out towards a grassy slope and the shade of the pines, and you can focus on this tranquil north woods landscape all day long. The park manager hopes to soon clear some of the nearby alder understory to provide views of a small nearby lake.

This is a bare-bones cabin: There's no electricity or heat,

and the nearest toilet is about 100 yards away in the campground (a bit farther to the restrooms and shower). However, drinking water is available right across the road. If you want minimalist camping with a roof, this is the place for you!

Crow Wing State Park is spread out along the beautiful forested banks of the Mississippi River right at its confluence with the Crow Wing River—offering twice the scenery, wildlife, paddling opportunities, and fishing you find in most parks.

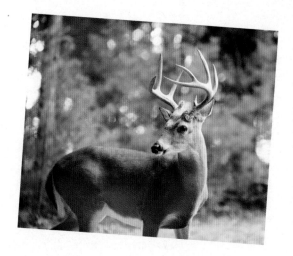

TOM'S TIPS: If you enjoy camping but want to kick it up a notch, this is the cabin for you. The setting is ideal, the campsite very spacious; because you have no cabin lights or heat source, you can still enjoy the challenge of "roughing it," albeit to a lesser extent.

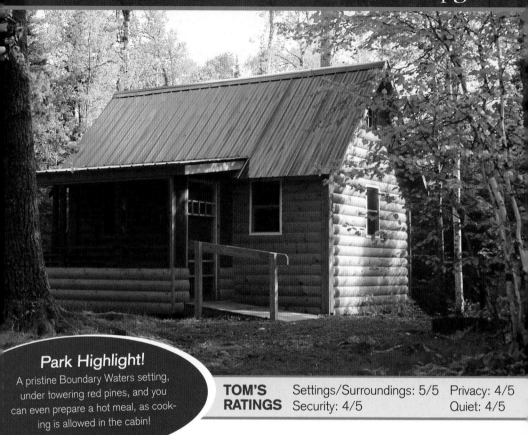

Park Highlight!

A pristine Boundary Waters setting, under towering red pines, and you can even prepare a hot meal, as cooking is allowed in the cabin!

TOM'S RATINGS Settings/Surroundings: 5/5 Privacy: 4/5
Security: 4/5 Quiet: 4/5

Number of cabins/availability: 3; seasonal (May–Oct.); check with Forest Service for opening dates.

Cabin sleeping capacity: *Alder:* 2 bunks, 1 bed, sleeps 5; *Tamarack* and *Aspen:* 2 bunks, 1 bed, and 2 additional beds in a loft; they sleep 7.

Cabin features: No electricity or heat. All cabins: ADA accessible (except for bunk beds), beds feature a countertop for cooking (must bring own equipment), foam mattresses, fire pits with grills, and a picnic table. *Alder* and *Aspen:* have roofed porches. *Tamarack:* features a screened porch.

Where to find water/bathrooms: Toilets are just a short walk from the *Alder* and *Aspen* cabins and adjacent to *Tamarack*; drinking water is accessible between *Alder* cabin and campsite 3.

Reservations/fees: You can make reservations through recreation.gov or you can make payments at nearby Bearskin Lodge (www.bearskin.com) $68/night.

Restrictions: Domestic pets are allowed; general campground rules are posted at site.

GPS: 48.038743, -90.400277

Key information: Bearskin Lodge (which runs the cabins), 124 E. Bearskin Road, Grand Marais, MN 55604, Bearskin Lodge: 800-338-4170, www.bearskin.com or www.recreation.gov

Area activities/attractions:

The campground includes a boat ramp and an entry point for the Boundary Waters Canoe Area Wilderness along the eastern half of the lake (permits required). The nearby Bearskin Lodge runs the cabins, in addition to the other cabins and campsites it oversees. The lodge also provides licenses, boat rentals, and carries an assortment of supplies.

Notes: These three national forest cabins add a touch of cozy, yet rustic, comfort to this portion of the northern lake country. Situated right at the western edge of the Boundary Waters Canoe Area Wilderness, all three cabins here are quite spacious, partly due to a slightly different floor plan than most every other camper cabin in the state. The entry door and porch are on the side of the cabin instead of at the end. Visually, this makes the cabin seem larger than others. *Alder* has the standard double bed and twin bunks common to most

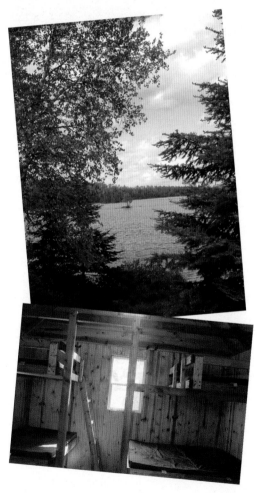

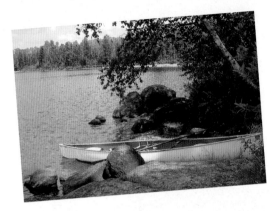

camper cabins, while *Tamarack* and *Alder* feature a ladder-accessible loft with a platform and a pad for two more sleepers.

Besides the extra sleeping space, you can cook in these cabins using a camp stove or other fuel-fed appliance. There is counter space to use as a makeshift kitchen, but with no electricity or water, you'll have to rely on your gas stove cooking skills. *Tamarack* is the newest of the three cabins here, and all are aligned along the numbered campsites in the small campground. Plans are underway for adding three more cabins too.

The cabins have ample space outside for fire rings and tables, and the huge pines provide a canopy of shade for each site. This is truly a north woods arena for a cabin. The lake is nearby and part of a chain of the long, narrow lakes common throughout the BWCA. Those familiar with the region can incorporate the nearby portages to Flour, Alder, and Crocodile Lakes when planning canoe routes, so a canoe trip can start just a few steps from these delightful cabins.

TOM'S TIPS: Each cabin has its own particular advantages: *Aspen* is closest to the lake, but *Alder* is closer to the boat dock and the drinking water is also nearby; *Tamarack* is the newest of the three, sleeps more people and is right next door to the toilets, but it's also the farthest from the lake. Together they provide a camping experience that is as much a part of the BWCA as paddling a canoe.

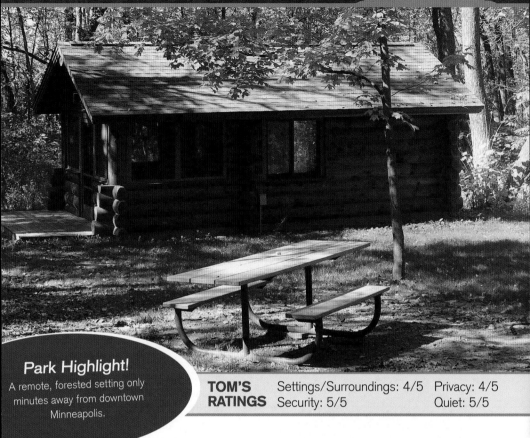

TOM'S RATINGS

Settings/Surroundings: 4/5 Privacy: 4/5
Security: 5/5 Quiet: 5/5

Number of cabins/availability: 2, seasonal (mid-May–mid-Oct.).

Cabin sleeping capacity: Cabin 1 sleeps 5 (ADA accessible); Cabin 2 sleeps 6.

Cabin features: Electricity and outlets, heat, ceiling fan, overhead lighting, table and benches, bunk beds, fire ring, picnic table, and a screened porch.

Where to find water/bathrooms: There is a drinking fountain at the end of the driveways that connect the cabins; there is a vault toilet in the parking lot.

Reservations/fees: Required. Call 763-559-6700; $60/night with a two-night minimum on weekends and holidays; there's a six-night maximum stay within any 30-day period.

Restrictions: No cooking, pets, or smoking.

GPS: Entrance to gated road to cabins, 45.188082, -93.437444

Key information: Elm Creek Park Reserve, 12400 James Deane Parkway, Maple Grove, MN 55369, 763-694-7894, www.threeriversparks.org/parks/elm-creek-park.aspx

Area activities/attractions: The attractions are mostly concentrated in the southern half of the park and include hiking, biking, archery, disc golf, picnic areas, and camping. Winter activities include cross-country skiing, snowshoeing, downhill skiing, sledding, snowboarding, and snowmobiling.

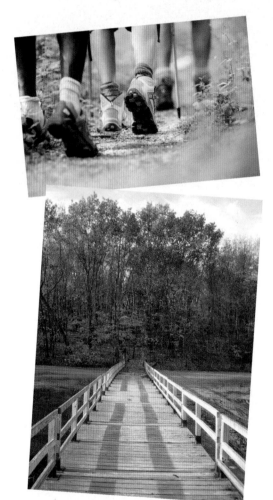

Notes: One of the western suburbs of Minneapolis, Maple Grove boasts the 4,900-acre Elm Creek Park Reserve, which is the largest park in the impressive Three Rivers Park District. Elm Creek features two rustic camper cabins, and they are situated all on their own.

To reach the cabins, you take a dirt road that leads south into the park. It then heads a short distance through lush woods, including a corridor of hardwoods, mostly maples. The road gently rises and dips, leading to the cabins at the end of the roadway, which is a drive of about 1/3 mile.

Each cabin has its own driveway, and the cabins are set off into the trees; nearby there's a clearing that features a parking area, a drinking fountain, and a vault toilet. About 150 feet of trees and shrubbery separate the two cabins giving each beautiful, private surroundings, and the cabins are mostly out of view of each other.

This wooded, northern section of Elm Creek is tucked away in a rustic area of the park that doesn't see too many intrusions beyond the traffic on the paved North Loop Trail. The cabins also have easy access to the 11-mile circuit that loops through the park. Cabin users have the option of hiking the unpaved Group Camp Trail that leads out into the open marshlands and grasses west of the cabins. The trail swings north through a treeless area before reentering the woods and linking back up to the dirt road just north of the cabins.

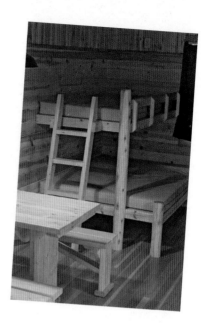

TOM'S TIPS: The lower region of the park, the hub of which is the Elm Creek Nature Center, features opportunities to enjoy archery, camping, disc golf, horse and mountain bike trails, a picnic area, and a swimming area. The extensive paved trail system leading out from the Nature Center crisscrosses through wooded areas along creeks and around small lakes, showcasing most of the entire southern section of this expansive park.

Park Highlight!

A sandy-bottomed swimming pool is just a short distance from two rustic wood cabins and a recently converted stone cottage.

TOM'S RATINGS
Settings/Surroundings: 3/5   Privacy: 2/5
Security: 3/5   Quiet: 3/5

Number of cabins/availability: 2; year-round. Cabins are available daily in summer, Thurs.–Sun. in winter.

Cabin sleeping capacity: *Hackberry Haven* sleeps 5 (ADA accessible); *Coffeetree Retreat* sleeps 6.

Cabin features: Electricity, heat, table and benches, bunk beds, fire ring, picnic table, and screened porch.

Where to find water/bathrooms: Water is located between cabins, just across campground road; showers and flush toilets are available seasonally and are just 350–400 feet away in the campground. Vault toilets are adjacent to *Hackberry Haven* cabin.

Reservations/fees: 866-857-2757; www.dnr.state.mn.us; Sun.–Thurs. $55/night; Fri.–Sat. $65/night.

Restrictions: No cooking, pets, or smoking.

GPS: Entrance to cabin/campground loop, 44.294725, -94.470172

Key information: Flandrau State Park, 1300 Summit Avenue, New Ulm, MN 56073, 507-233-9800, www.dnr.state.mn.us/state_parks/flandrau/index.html

Area activities/attractions: The park has a chlorinated, sandy-bottom swimming pool (open Memorial Day–mid-Aug.) and a seasonal beach house and group center, all of which are ADA accessible. The park also has a playground with volleyball/horseshoes, 8 miles of hiking trails, 6 miles of cross-country skiing trails, and 2 miles of groomed snowshoe trails. The park also allows hosts a limited bowhunting season each year. Supplies and services are available in nearby New Ulm.

Notes: The cabins are situated along the outer loop of the non-electric section of the campground, along the base of a steep, treelined slope. Both cabins are set back from the road beyond a grassy front yard that separates them from tent campsites over in the campground. Like most cabin sites located within the campground loop, the amount of privacy and solitude you'll enjoy depends mostly on the number of nearby campers. *Hackberry Haven* is closest to the vault toilet, and you'll need to take a short walk to reach the showers, which are located between the campground loops.

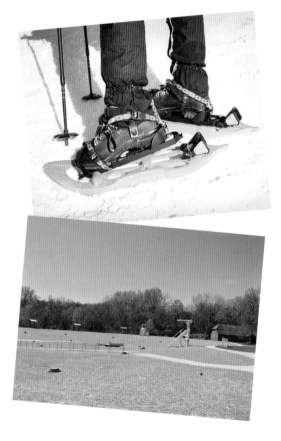

Flandrau State Park is situated on the eastern edge of the state's prairie region in west-central Minnesota. The park, located immediately adjacent to the City of New Ulm, is a landscape of river bottomlands accented with massive cottonwood trees, steep riverbanks, and networked with trails for both summer and winter use.

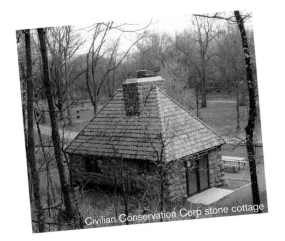

Civilian Conservation Corp stone cottage

The Cottonwood River flows through the park, and the Dakota Indians first inhabited the area. It was later visited by French explorers and eventually converted into farmland. During World War II, Flandrau was the site of a POW site for captured Germans. The WPA-era building on site now serves as the park's Group Center.

Another physical reminder of the park's history is the Civilian Conservation Corp stone cottage, which is located next to the cabins.

TOM'S TIPS: Clearly the coolest feature of this park is the huge outdoor, sandy-beached swimming "pool." Located within a short walk of all the campground loops, it's open from Memorial Day through mid-August attracting residents from town as well as visiting campers. Much of this state park consists of open lowlands that lack trails, making it especially inviting to explore via snowshoe in the winter.

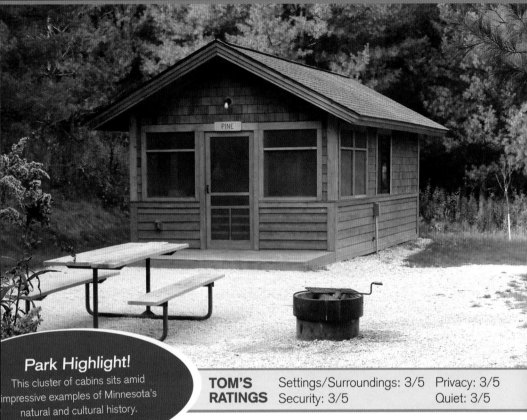

Park Highlight!
This cluster of cabins sits amid impressive examples of Minnesota's natural and cultural history.

TOM'S RATINGS

Settings/Surroundings: 3/5   Privacy: 3/5
Security: 3/5   Quiet: 3/5

Number of cabins/availability: 5; year-round.

Cabin sleeping capacity: *Pine, Mink, Owl:* 6; *Lily, Trout:* 5 (ADA accessible).

Cabin features: Electricity, heat, table and seating, bunk beds, overhead bed lights, wall hooks, fire ring, and a picnic table.

Where to find water/bathrooms: Water and a vault toilet are available in each cabin cluster. Showers and restrooms are available seasonally nearby between campground Loops B and C. The picnic shelter complex is open year-round and has restrooms and water.

Reservations/fees: 866-857-2757; www.dnr.state.mn.us; Sun.–Thurs. $60/night; Fri.–Sat. $70/night.

Restrictions: No cooking, pets, or smoking. Note: There are special restrictions for cave tours (inquire when making reservations).

GPS: Entrance to campground area: 43.633698, -92.225769; Entrance to cabin complex: 43.627929, -92.221689

Key information: Forestville State Park, 21071 County 118, Preston, MN 55965, 507-352-5111, forestville.statepark@state.mn.us, www.dnr.state.mn.us/state_parks/forestville_mystery_cave/index.html

Area activities/attractions: The park features hiking, trout fishing, camping, historic village tours, a variety of caving tours, groomed cross-country skiing, and snowmobiling.

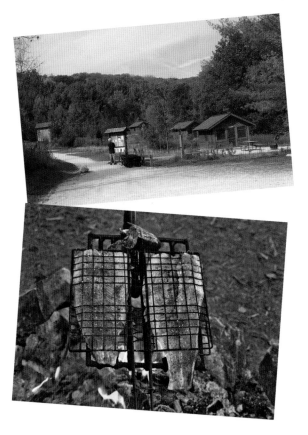

Notes: The setting for the cabins at Forestville merely hints at the wealth of attractions in this park. All five "walk-in" units are situated along a broad gravel walkway off a large parking lot. Camping carts make hauling gear to each unit easy. The *Lily, Mink,* and *Trout* cabins are each set off the trail towards the edge of a hardwood-conifer forest that flanks the entire cabin complex. *Owl* and *Pine* are tucked back into the understory along a knoll that rises slightly above the other cabins.

Surrounded by a light understory and a scattering of pines and a few mixed hardwoods, *Pine* is the most secluded of the five. *Owl* has a commanding and slightly lofty view down to the walk-in entrance. *Lily, Mink,* and *Trout* each have their own spacious sites that afford cabin guests more privacy. *Trout*, one of two ADA accessible cabins, faces directly towards the parking lot at the head of the walk-in trail.

Amenities and attractions abound throughout the park, and they make this cabin experience even more appealing. After a day of adventuring along the 19 miles of trails here (some of which ascend over 200 feet in elevation), fishing in the blue ribbon trout streams, walking through an 1880s-era frontier village, or exploring Minnesota's longest known cave (perhaps spelunking on your belly with flashlight in hand), a soothing evening in a cabin is just the ticket.

TOM'S TIPS: These cabins aren't far from Mystery Cave, which is Minnesota's longest known cave. It has year-round temperature of 48°F, and visitors can take a variety of "cool" tours (including the ever-popular "scenic tour") or specialized tours (such as a flashlight tour, a geology tour, photography tours, or wild caving tours). For history buffs, Historic Forestville offers an authentic re-creation of a once-thriving town circa the late 1800s.

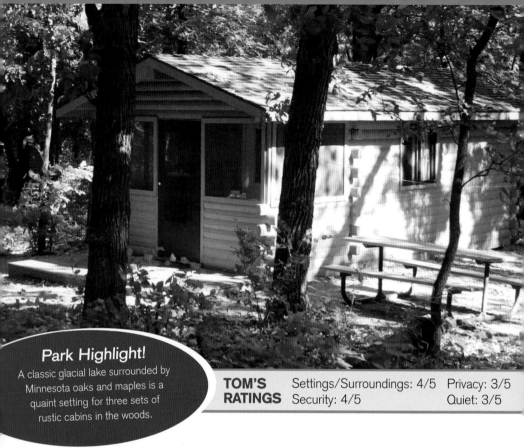

TOM'S RATINGS

Settings/Surroundings: 4/5   Privacy: 3/5
Security: 4/5   Quiet: 3/5

Number of cabins/availability: 6; 2 seasonal, 4 year-round. *Friends* and *Coneflower* (wheelchair accessible) are available Apr.–Labor Day. *Kettle, Kame, Glacial Erratic,* and *Esker* are available year-round.

Cabin sleeping capacity: Seasonal cabins: *Friends* sleeps 6; *Coneflower* sleeps 5; **Year-round cabins:** *Kettle, Glacial Erratic,* and *Kame* sleep 6; *Esker* sleeps 5.

Cabin features: Seasonal cabins: No electricity or heat, table and seating, bunk beds, fire ring, and picnic table. *Coneflower* is wheelchair accessible; **Year-round cabins:** electricity, heat, table and seating, and bunk beds. *Esker* and *Glacier* have ceiling fans. *Esker* is wheelchair accessible.

Where to find water/bathrooms: A vault toilet and a frost-free drinking water outlet are available outside the park office year-round. In the summer, there are restrooms at the beach (but no showers); these are located near the parking lot between the four year-round cabins. A modern, seasonally available restroom/shower facility is located near the center of the lower campground loop.

Reservations/fees: 866-857-2757; www.dnr.state.mn.us; Sun.–Thurs. $60/night; Fri.–Sat. $70/night.

Restrictions: No cooking, pets, or smoking.

GPS: Entrance to *Kettle/Kames* cabins, 45.540865, -95.526798; entrance to *Esker/Glacial Erractic*, 45.540674, -95.524618; entrance to *Coneflower/Friends*, 45.540674, -95.524618

Key information: Glacial Lakes State Park, 25022 County Road 41, Starbuck, MN 56381, 320-239-2860, www.dnr.state.mn.us/state_parks/glacial_lakes/index.html

During the off-season, contact: Lake Carlos State Park Office, 2601 County Road 38 NE, Carlos, MN 56319, 320-852-7200

Area activities/attractions:
The park is home to extensive naturalist programs, hiking and horseback trails, paddling (including rentals of boats, canoes, kayaks, and stand-up paddleboards, as well as fishing, swimming, snowshoeing, and cross-country skiing. There are also numerous lakes in the region, and fishing for northern, walleye, crappie, and perch is popular. There's also a 4-mile bike trail to nearby Starbuck, and there are numerous specialty shops in communities throughout the Central Lakes area north of the park.

Notes: Three sets of side-by-side cabins are at distinct locations around Signaless Lake, a glacial lake with 50-plus acres of clear

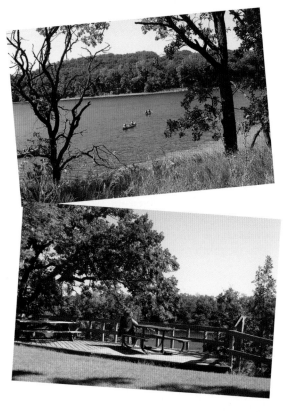

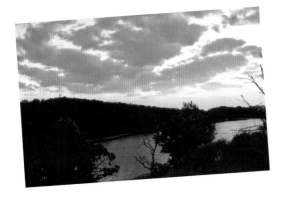

water. The entire drainage/watershed lies within the boundaries of the park, so no matter which cabins you stay in, the natural amenities of this park are close at hand.

Glacial Lakes State Park is one of only a few with cabins spread throughout the park instead of being clustered all in one area. Each pair of units is in a unique setting that captures an aspect of the park right out the front door.

The *Kettle* and *Kame* cabins are perched on a hill overlooking the boat landing and fishing pier, and both cabins hold a commanding view of the northwestern end of Signaless Lake. *Kame* cabin is tucked back into the treeline, giving it more shade and perhaps a bit more privacy than the neighboring *Kettle* cabin.

Esker and the *Glacial Erratic* cabin are surrounded by a mature stand of bur oaks and other hardwoods, and each cabin faces slightly towards the other, making them especially suitable for a double cabin outing with friends. They don't have a lake view, however.

Coneflower and *Friends* cabins are located next to the lower campground, and these two seasonal cabins are at the edge of the hardwood forests that blanket the hills overlooking the northern end of Signaless Lake.

TOM'S TIPS: A 0.8-mile self-guided interpretive trail leads south out from Oakridge Campground, and the trail follows along above the shore of Signaless Lake and continues to the group camp parking area where hikers can connect up with the park's network of hiking and equestrian trails. Bicyclists and hikers can also head out on the bike trail that connects the park entrance to the city of Starbuck, 4 miles to the north.

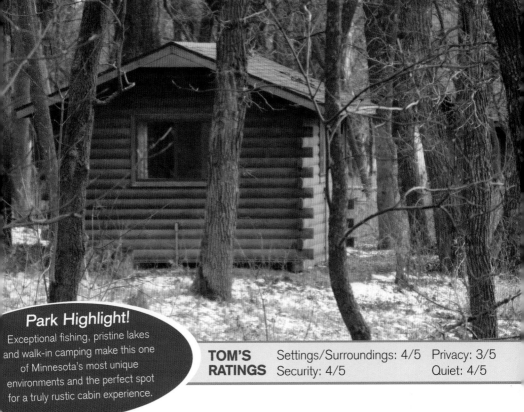

Park Highlight!
Exceptional fishing, pristine lakes and walk-in camping make this one of Minnesota's most unique environments and the perfect spot for a truly rustic cabin experience.

TOM'S RATINGS Settings/Surroundings: 4/5   Privacy: 3/5
Security: 4/5   Quiet: 4/5

Number of cabins/availability: 4, plus 2 camper yurts; year-round.

Cabin sleeping capacity: Cabin 1 sleeps 5 and is ADA accessible; Cabins 2–4 sleep 6; the *Eagle* yurt sleeps 7; the *Osprey* yurt sleeps 3.

Cabin features: Cabin: Electricity, propane "fireplace" heater, table/benches, bunk beds, fire ring, picnic table, and screened porch; **Yurts:** No electricity; indoor woodstove, table and chairs, and bunk beds.

Where to find water/bathrooms: Showers, restrooms, and water are all available seasonally in the restroom building at the campground entrance.

Reservations/fees: 866-857-2757; dnr.state.mn.us
  Cabins: Sun.–Thurs. $60/night; Fri.–Sat. $70/night
  Yurts: 7-person yurt: Sun.–Thurs. $60/night; Fri.–Sat. $65/night
      3-person yurt: Sun.–Thurs. $50/night; Fri.–Sat. $60/night

Restrictions: No cooking, pets, or smoking.

GPS: Entrance to walk-in cabins/campground, 46.328160, -95.668854

Key information: Glendalough State Park, 25287 Whitetail Lane, Battle Lake, MN 56515, 218-864-0110, www.dnr.state.mn.us/state_parks/glendalough/index.html

Area activities/attractions: The park has nearly 20 miles of assorted biking and hiking trails, 7 miles of groomed cross-country skiing trails, and 1.5 miles of groomed snowshoeing trails; there's also many canoeing opportunities on the park's chain of lakes, fishing (including large and plentiful panfish), a fishing pier, remote tent camping, a sandy swimming beach, and a broad range of rental equipment for both summer and winter.

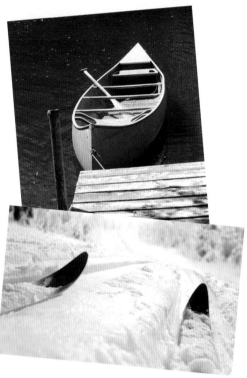

Notes: The four cabins are located within the wooded loop of the walk-in campground, and each is nestled in among the hardwood understory with plenty of vegetation to provide some privacy.

The entrance hub of the walk-in campground includes the restroom and shower facilities as well as an info kiosk and the access point for firewood and water. An overstory of maples and oaks provides a shady canopy for the campground and cabins.

The cabin sites, like the campsites nearby, are all part of the "walk-in" community at Glendalough. And because the cabins are located in a campground, the surrounding attractions and natural amenities are all close at hand.

In all, the park covers nearly 2,000 acres of land and has an incredible 1,000 acres of water between its six lakes. The lakes in the park feature more than 9.2 miles of undeveloped shoreline, one of the largest (and last) such tracts in western Minnesota. Lake Emma features two observation decks and a floating observation blind. Trails loop among the lakes and tie them all together within the park.

In August, there's a special treat—several hundred monarch butterflies fly through on their southward migration.

TOM'S TIPS: Probably the most unique aspect of this park is the fisheries management of Annie Battle Lake. Once a summer retreat and then a game farm, it has experienced relatively little fishing pressure. This history, coupled with specific regulations, has fostered a population of incredibly huge crappies and bluegills. (There's also a special fishing regulation for the lake, with a limit

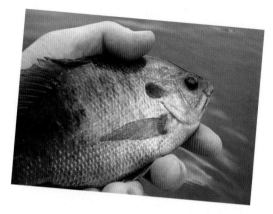

of 5 bluegills/crappies per day.) If you're up for an adventure, Glendalough also has two remote yurts, accessible on foot or by boat, on the far side of Annie Battle Lake.

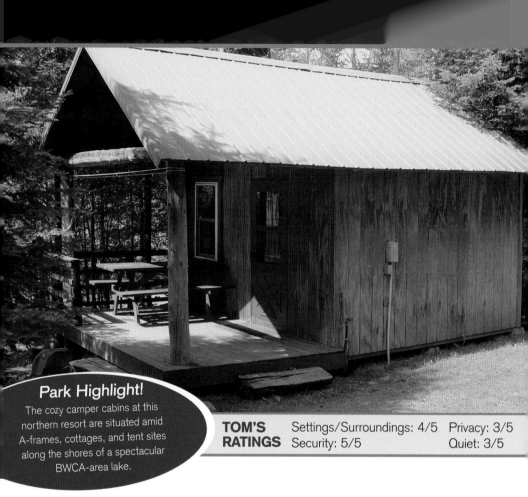

Park Highlight!
The cozy camper cabins at this northern resort are situated amid A-frames, cottages, and tent sites along the shores of a spectacular BWCA-area lake.

TOM'S RATINGS

Settings/Surroundings: 4/5   Privacy: 3/5
Security: 5/5   Quiet: 3/5

Number of cabins/availability: 3; seasonal (early May–early Oct.).

Cabin sleeping capacity: 5

Cabin features: Electricity, two chairs, 2 sets of bunk beds (the upper beds are twin beds; the lower beds are double beds), a 4-foot counter with a cupboard area, fire ring, picnic table on porch, a covered porch, and a main lodge with sitting area and store/gift shop, with snacks and supplies.

Where to find water/bathrooms: Restrooms and showers are available in the campground shower house adjacent to Camper Cabin 18 (across the road from cabins 19 and 20). Water is also available nearby.

Reservations/fees: (800) 533-5814; www.gunflintpines.com/reserve.shtml
Early May–mid June: $57/midweek; $67/Fri.–Sat.; Mid June–early Sept.: $75/night;

Early Sept.–early Oct.: $57/midweek; $67/Fri.–Sat.; a 30 percent deposit is required at time of booking; there are also fees for additional adults/kids.

Restrictions: No cooking or smoking in cabins; pets are allowed, but must be on a leash.

GPS: 48.087173, -90.741927

Key information: Gunflint Pines Resort & Campground, 217 South Gunflint Lake Road, Grand Marais, MN 55604, 218-388-4454 (no cell service beyond Grand Marais), www.gunflintpines.com

Notes: Yes, this is technically a private resort, but the cabins and campground are very much reminiscent of a state park, but one located in the middle of lake country right on the cusp of the spectacular Boundary Waters. The three cabins here are nestled into wooded openings along the campground loop, not in a simple line, like a lakeside motel as seen at most other resort cabins.

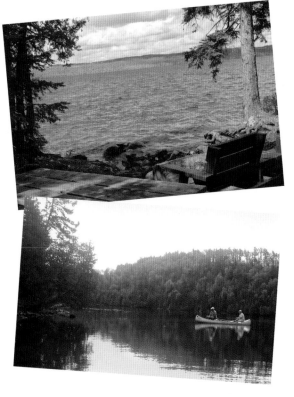

The cabins here are pretty basic when it comes to looks and furnishings, but they provide that one step up for those who don't want to tent camp. Unlike many camper cabins, there isn't a table or chair inside; instead, the cabins come with two chairs and a picnic table right outside the front door on the porch. Of course, you can always bring your own camp table/chairs to complement the interior counter space.

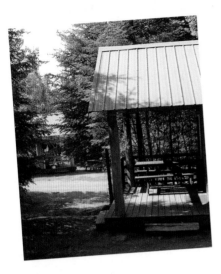

The cabins' real appeal lies in their location on Gunflint Lake, which is long, narrow, and lined with birch and evergreens. It's also less than a mile from Canada. Although the cabins back up into a wooded area, it's a very short walk down to the shaded shoreline, and the view across the sky-blue waters is incredible.

When you visit, you can bring your cell phone along, but don't expect to use it while this far north. There's no reception beyond Grand Marias on the Lake Superior shoreline. But who cares? Talk to Mother Nature instead. Go hiking, spend hours fishing or taking pictures of wildlife, or, if you're lucky, even see the northern lights.

TOM'S TIPS: The resort is a very friendly and easy going place, especially the main lodge where you can relax with an ice-cream cone or delightful root beer. The cabins are close to the lodge but set just enough back to offer a North Woods feel within the "resort" setting.

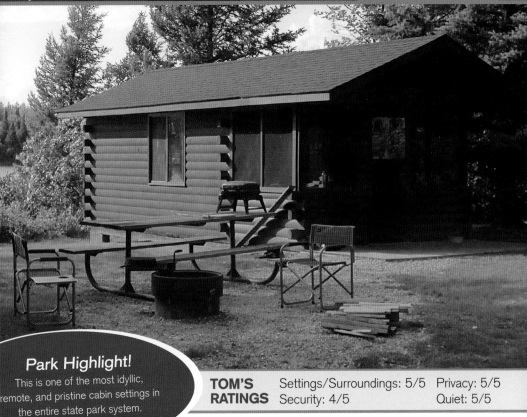

Park Highlight!
This is one of the most idyllic, remote, and pristine cabin settings in the entire state park system.

TOM'S RATINGS   Settings/Surroundings: 5/5   Privacy: 5/5
Security: 4/5   Quiet: 5/5

Number of cabins/availability: 2; seasonal (typically May 1–Oct. 31).

Cabin sleeping capacity: 6

Cabin features: *Timberline Cabin:* Electricity, space heater, table and seating, bunk beds, and screened porch; *Camp 3:* No electricity or heat; table and seating, bunk beds, and screened porch.

Where to find water/bathrooms: *Timberline Cabin:* Water and restrooms are nearby within the campground loop; *Camp 3 Cabin:* There is a vault toilet at the cabin site but no water on site; the nearest restroom and shower facilities are available seasonally at the campground.

Reservations/fees: 866-857-2757; dnr.state.mn.us
    Camp 3 Cabin (no electricity/heat): Sun.–Thurs. $55/night; Fri.–Sat. $65/night
    Timberline Cabin (has electricity/heat): Sun.–Thurs. $60/night; Fri.–Sat. $70/night

Restrictions: No cooking, pets, or smoking.

GPS: Entrance to park, 48.643904, -95.545180; location of *Camp 3 Cabin*, 48.625839, -95.526676

Key information: Hayes Lake State Park, 48990 Country Road 4, Roseau, MN 56751, 218-425-7504, www.dnr.state.mn.us/state_parks/hayes_lake/index.html

Off-season contact: Lake Bronson State Park, 218-754-2200

Area activities/attractions: Swimming, fishing, and paddling are ever-popular in the lake; canoe, kayak, and rowboat rentals are available, as are electric trolling motors and batteries (no gas motors are allowed on the lake). The park also has 13 miles of hiking trails, 5 miles of mountain bike trails, and 7 miles of equestrian trails. In the winter, visitors enjoy the 9 miles of snowmobile trails and 11 miles of groomed cross-country ski trails.

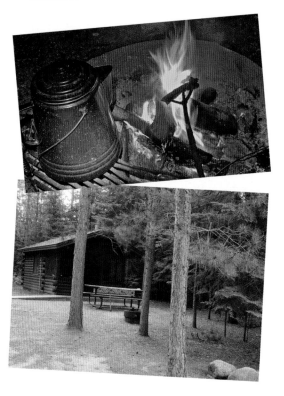

Notes: The cabin settings at Hayes Lake are as different as night and day. *Timberline Cabin* is nestled into a modest stand of red pine at the far end of the shorter of the two campground loops. It's set back from the road and just off the trail that leads to the Bog Walk and observation points along nearby Hayes Lake. It's a spacious setting within the 30-plus campsites in this campground.

Then there's the cabin at *Camp 3*. It's located towards the southern arm of the lake, halfway between the main campground and the really remote group camp. To get to it, you have to literally head down a narrow, shrub-lined, 1.5-mile corridor along a rugged forest road that passes through dense stands of hardwoods. It's slow-going but a rewarding journey.

Camp 3 sits in a large, open clearing flanked by shrubs within the northern forest and overlooking the lower arm of Hayes Lake. The cabin faces towards the center of the clearing, which makes it easier to haul in gear from the parking area. Both the view from the clearing and the back window of the cabin look out over the lake. Once you take it all in, you find 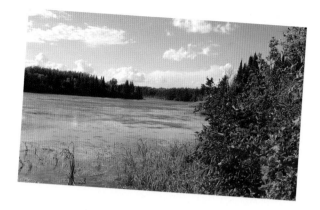 yourself in a pristine, remote North Woods setting. There's no campground noise, no road traffic, and jet skis and speedboats won't bother you, as only electric motors are allowed on the lake. This makes *Camp 3 Cabin* one of the most peaceful and inviting cabins in the entirety of the state park system.

TOM'S TIPS: Canoeing and kayaking are popular here, and anglers can seek out crappies, sunfish, largemouth bass, and northern pike in the lake, which was formed when the North Fork of the Roseau River was dammed.

Park Highlight!

These camper cabins are brand new and in a great location, as they're situated along the Mississippi River on the shores of Lake Pepin.

TOM'S RATINGS

Settings/Surroundings: 4/5   Privacy: 4/5
Security: 5/5   Quiet: 5/5

Number of cabins/availability: 3, all of which are named for boats that once sailed on Lake Pepin: *Steamer Capital, Steamer Avalon*, and *J.S. De Luxe*; seasonal (May–mid-Oct.).

Cabin sleeping capacity: 6

Cabin features: Electricity, heat, table and benches, a large 16' x 24' floor plan, 2 sets of bunk beds with mattresses (the lower are queen-sized; the upper are twin beds), air-conditioning, fire ring, picnic table, all cabins are ADA accessible, open porch with a light, and a large set-back front yard.

Where to find water/bathrooms: The *Steamer Avalon* cabin is closest to the modern bathhouse; *Steamer Capital* cabin is set farthest back from the road. Drinking water is available across from the *Steamer Capital* cabin. A vault toilet is not far from the *J.S. De Luxe* cabin.

Reservations/fees: 651-345-3855; hoksila@ci.lake-city.mn.us Security deposit is $100. Contact the campground for current rates.

Restrictions: No cooking, no pets, no tents allowed on cabin site; no vehicle parking at cabins; parking is available nearby, however.

GPS: Entrance off of U.S. Hwy 61, 2 miles north of Lake City, 44.469217, -92.296544

Key information: Hok-Si-La Municipal Park and Campground, 2500 N. Highway 61 Boulevard, Lake City, MN 55041, 651-345-3855, www.hoksilapark.org

Area activities/attractions: There are also screened shelters nearby, an Education and Interpretive Center in the main campground complex, a swimming beach, river access and a boat launch, volleyball and basketball courts, and nature trails. The park store offers limited supplies and ice; full services and supplies are available in nearby Lake City.

Notes: Recently built, these three cabins are part of a unique campground arrangement: no cars at the campsites! Campers and cabin guests can drive in, unload, and then drive back out to the parking area outside the campground complex. It's a short walk, but there's a definite benefit: You'll only hear the faint sounds of foot traffic in this riverside setting.

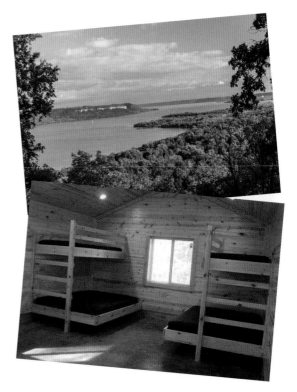

Located along the Minnesotan shores of Lake Pepin, a 1.7-mile wide stretch of the mighty Mississippi River, the park offers lowland forests of massive cottonwoods, lots of riverfront (and the water activities that go with it), and a commanding view of the river bluffs on the Wisconsin side of this great river.

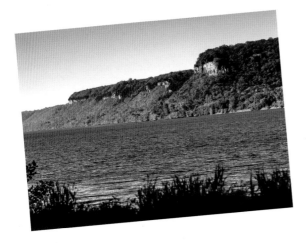

Birding is one of the more popular pastimes at the park, and hikers enjoy observing the shorebirds along the network of trails that follow the park's mile of shoreline. Like the park's tent sites, which are laid out within several loops along the road network, the cabin sites are very spacious with huge front lawns. Inside, the cabins are equally roomy; these are some of the largest camper cabins in the state.

This section of the Mississippi River is generally a tranquil body of water and ideal for swimming (there's a swimming beach but no lifeguard) and paddle sports (a large boat access area is immediately north of the campground complex).

When you approach Hok-Si-La for the first time it may appear to be an outdoor camp compound, but the friendly staff, roomy sites, and river frontage all come together to form a unique camping experience along the banks of this iconic river.

TOM'S TIPS: While you can stock up your cabin with carloads of gear, plan on bringing your walking shoes and enjoy the laid-back ambiance of this quiet, woody park that encourages you to slow down and enjoy the quieter moments.

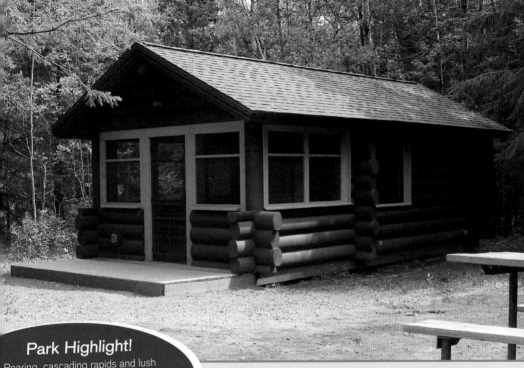

Park Highlight!
Roaring, cascading rapids and lush northern forests provide an inviting backdrop for the cabins in this popular northern Minnesota park.

TOM'S RATINGS

Settings/Surroundings: 4/5   Privacy: 4/5
Security: 4/5   Quiet: 3/5

Number of cabins/availability: 5; year-round.

Cabin sleeping capacity: *Slate, Gabbro*, and *Shale* sleep 6; *Agate* and *Basalt* sleep 5 and are ADA accessible.

Cabin features: Electricity, heat, table and benches, bunk beds, fire ring, picnic table, and screened porch.

Where to find water/bathrooms: Water is available in the campground loop across the road from the *Basalt* cabin (near campsite 57) and at the outside faucets near the River Inn. Two frost-free hydrants are available year-round at the campground and another is located between the park office and River Inn.

Water and toilets are also adjacent to the *Agate, Gabbro*, and *Shale* cabin sites; restrooms and showers for all cabins are centrally located on the main road near the campground hub. Water, restrooms, and showers close for the season in mid-October.

Reservations/fees: 866-857-2757; www.dnr.state.mn.us; Sun.–Thurs. $60/night; Fri.–Sat. $70/night.

Restrictions: No cooking, pets, or smoking.

GPS: Campground entrance, 46.655312, -92.372794

Key information: Jay Cooke State Park, 780 Highway 210, Carlton, MN 55718, 218-673-7000, www.dnr.state.mn.us/state_parks/jay_cooke/index.html

Area activities/attractions: Amenities at the park include 50 miles of hiking trails, 12 miles of snowmobile trails, 32 miles of cross-country ski trails, along with scenic attractions including the famous Swinging Bridge, the Thompson Dam, and river gorge, as well as the Grand Portage Trail and the Munger State Trail.

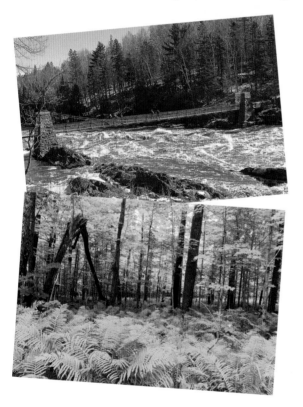

Notes: The cabins here provide casual, comfortable accommodations amid one of Minnesota's most ruggedly scenic state parks. Two of the park's cabins, *Basalt* and *Slate*, are located at the north end of a campground loop at the northern end of the park; the other three cabins, *Shale, Gabbro*, and *Agate*, are located off the main campground loop.

Tucked away in the northern part of the park, *Basalt* and *Slate* offer spacious, private sites surrounded by forest and rock outcroppings. The fire ring and picnic area for these cabins are also situated off to the side, hidden from road traffic by trees and understory. The trade-off for this semi-seclusion is a long jaunt to the restrooms and showers at the heart of the campground.

The three cabins near the main campground are in more open and exposed sites, and they are a little less private.

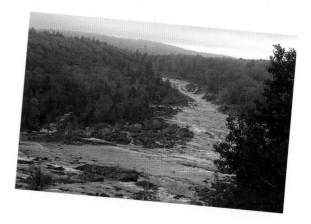

All five cabins are across the highway from a hardscrabble network of trails that looks down upon the raging St. Louis River below. The park's Swinging Bridge is a famous landmark and offers a stunning bird's-eye view of the cascading rapids. This steel suspension bridge free to "swing" on its cables makes the experience of waltzing over the roiling river beneath worth a trip to this park by itself. Couple that with a comfy cabin roost after a day of adventurous hiking—or skiing—and these cabins become even more appealing.

TOM'S TIPS: There are more than 50 miles of hiking trails throughout the park, as well as access to the Grand Portage Trail and the Willard Munger State Trail. Be sure to bring sturdy hiking boots, as the trails within the park are steep and rocky.

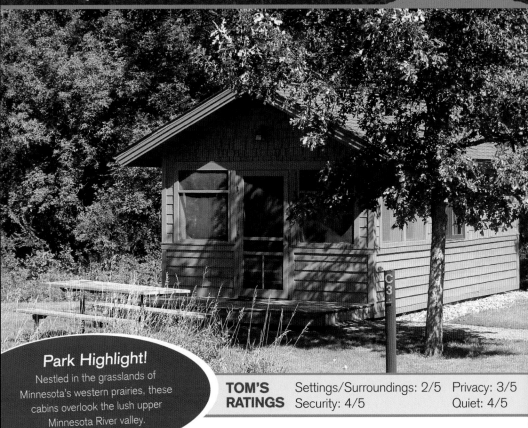

Park Highlight!

Nestled in the grasslands of Minnesota's western prairies, these cabins overlook the lush upper Minnesota River valley.

TOM'S RATINGS Settings/Surroundings: 2/5 Privacy: 3/5
Security: 4/5 Quiet: 4/5

Number of cabins/availability: 3; open year-round.

Cabin sleeping capacity: Cabins 1 and 3 sleep 6; Cabin 2 sleeps 5 and is wheelchair accessible.

Cabin features: Electricity, heat, air-conditioning, a ceiling fan, table and chairs, and screened porch.

Where to find water/bathrooms: A vault toilet is located within 200-300 feet of the cabins; a restroom and showers are available seasonally at the nearby adjacent campground; drinking water is located just beyond the cabins at the walk-in parking lot and seasonally at the main campground restroom.

Reservations/fees: 866-857-2757; www.dnr.state.mn.us; Sun.–Thurs. $60/night; Fri.–Sat. $70/night.

Restrictions: No cooking, pets, or smoking.

GPS: Entrance to park/campground, 45.044298, -95.878951

Key information: Lac Qui Parle State Park, 14047 20th Street NW, Watson, MN 56295, 320-734-4450, www.dnr.state.mn.us/state_parks/lac_qui_parle

Area activities/attractions: Fishing, hiking, wildlife viewing, canoeing, and kayaking, cross-country skiing, incredible bird-watching (especially during fall migration), the former site of Fort Renville, and the reconstructed Lac Qui Parle Mission building.

Notes: These three camper cabins are nestled into the golden prairie grasses on the edge of Lac Qui Parle, a reservoir created when the Minnesota River was dammed. The cabins here are located in the state park's upper campground area, which caters mainly to RV-style camping. Cabins 1 and 3 sit at the edge of a grove of mixed hardwoods bordering a grassy meadow. Cabin 2 is nestled atop the edge of the ancient valley rim and offers a sweeping view of the wooded river lowlands and lake below.

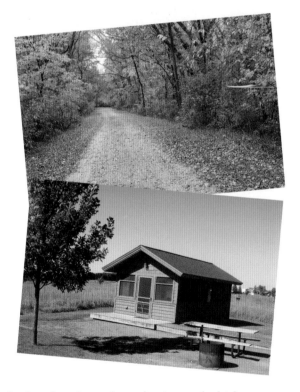

A hiking trail south from the cabins heads along a slope above the wooded shores of the lake and joins the highway near the site of Fort Renville, once a fur trading hub in the area. Today nothing remains of the site, but there is much nearby. Across the highway from the fort site overlook is a trail leading up over the hill to the state's largest living cottonwood tree, which is 106 feet tall. A bit farther south is the Lac Qui Parle Mission, where the first Dakota dictionary, grammar book, and gospel were translated.

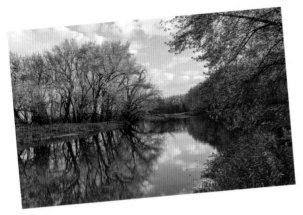

Fishing here is very popular in the summer, but the lake's also a great spot to check out during the winter, as it's not uncommon to see bald eagles out on the ice and perhaps even a coyote or fox romping over the frozen surface of Lac Qui Parle Lake.

The cabins here are "shade challenged" and are therefore the only camper-style cabins with air-conditioning in Minnesota's entire state park cabin network, something definitely to keep in mind if you want to avoid the hot, sticky days of summer camping.

TOM'S TIPS: Lac Qui Parle's lower campground has a network of grass-surfaced trails that wind through a river bottom landscape of lush grasses and towering cottonwoods and other deciduous trees. Deer abound in this park. A large variety of birds reside or travel through the park, including several species of owls, pileated woodpeckers, bald eagles, white pelicans and, of course, the thousands of geese and other waterfowl that visit during the migration season.

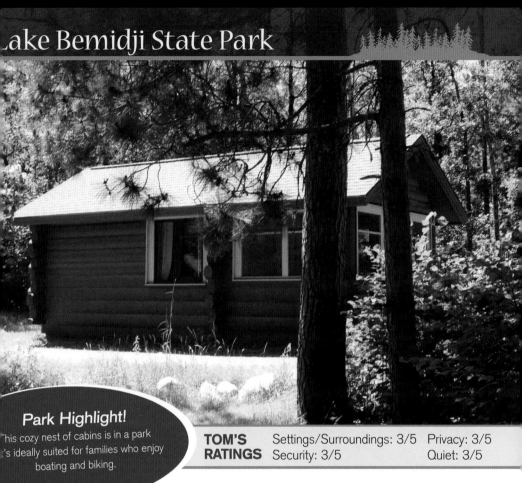

Park Highlight!
This cozy nest of cabins is in a park 's ideally suited for families who enjoy boating and biking.

TOM'S RATINGS

Settings/Surroundings: 3/5   Privacy: 3/5
Security: 3/5   Quiet: 3/5

Number of cabins/availability: 4; year-round.

Cabin sleeping capacity: *Tamarack* and *Maple* sleep 5 (ADA accessible); *Spruce* and *Balsam* sleep 6.

Cabin features: Electricity, heat, table and seating, bunk beds, fireplace, picnic table and screened porch.

Where to find water/bathrooms: Drinking water is available seasonally (early May–mid-October) between *Spruce* and *Tamarack* cabins and between *Balsam* and *Maple* cabins. Water is also available year-round at the Visitor Center. There are vault toilets year-round at the cabins and available restrooms year-round at the Visitor Center. Restrooms and showers also available seasonally in nearby Aspen Lane campground.

Reservations/fees: 866-857-2757; www.dnr.state.mn.us; Sun.–Thurs. $60/night; Fri.–Sat. $70/night.

Restrictions: No cooking, pets, or smoking.

GPS: Entrance to park, 47.540558, -94.835839; cabins area, 47.537979, -94.826191

Key information: Lake Bemidji State Park, 3401 State Park Road NE, Bemidji, MN 56601, 218-308-2300, www.dnr.state.mn.us/state_parks/lake_bemidji/index.html

Area activities/attractions: The park is home to 11 miles of hiking trails, 1.3 miles of bike trails, and 5 miles of mountain bike trails. Also, the northern trailhead for the 123-mile-long Paul Bunyan State Trail begins in Lake Bemidji State Park, and a portion of the trail joins the Heartland State Trail. If you don't have a bike, a "Nice Bike" rental service is operated in the park seasonally.

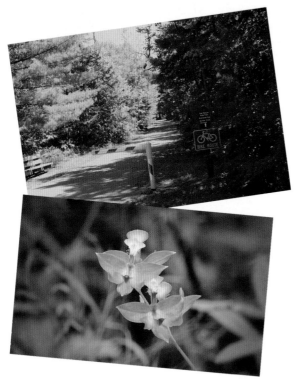

Other activities include swimming and paddling (rental canoes, kayaks, fishing boats are available), volleyball, and year-round naturalist programs. In the winter, the park offers 3 miles of snowmobiling trails, 8 miles of cross-country skiing trails, and snowshoeing (and rental gear).

Notes: These cabins are tucked in beneath a canopy of hardwoods and red pine trees and other conifers. *Spruce* and *Tamarack* are located on the north end of the cabin driveway loop while *Balsam* and *Maple* are situated off the southern end. Each has its own driveway, parking area, and a path for the very short walk to each cabin. Although the cabins are within earshot of each other, they each are situated to give a little privacy and a bit of yard space. The cabins are adjacent to the campground across the road but placed in a more rustic setting.

A highlight of the park's trail system is the 0.4-mile boardwalk at Big Bog Lake. Here you'll find insect-eating sundew plants and rare orchids thriving in a spruce-tamarack bog. Wildflower enthusiasts will enjoy searching for other rare finds, including pitcher plants, dragon's mouth, and showy lady slippers. Birders will be treated to a variety of warblers, vireos, and other forest songbirds as well as loons, terns, and perchance even an osprey along the shoreline of Lake Bemidji.

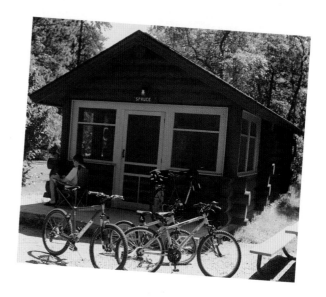

First and foremost, however, the cabins at Lake Bemidji State Park are ideally suited for the adventurous family that enjoys spending time on the trail and the lake, so if that's your family, head here!

TOM'S TIPS: The cabins are also a short bike ride or walk along the paved park roads to the northern trailhead of Paul Bunyan State Trail. Perfect for biking or hiking, its 123-mile-long route starts just beyond the park's boat ramp. And if you're looking for a place to store your gear, the cabins have plenty of room just outside the front door (or on the porch) to store several bikes or other adventuring items.

Lake Carlos State Park

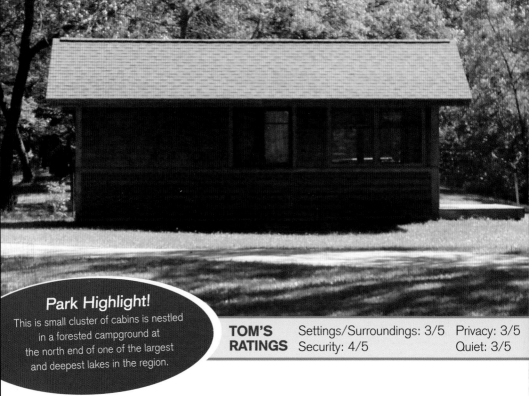

Park Highlight!
This is small cluster of cabins is nestled in a forested campground at the north end of one of the largest and deepest lakes in the region.

TOM'S RATINGS
Settings/Surroundings: 3/5   Privacy: 3/5
Security: 4/5   Quiet: 3/5

Number of cabins/availability: 4; year-round.

Cabin sleeping capacity: *Raccoon Hollow, Loon Nest,* and *Eagle Aerie* sleep 6; *Frog Pond* sleeps 5 (wheelchair accessible).

Cabin features: Electricity, heat, ceiling fan, table and seating, bunk beds, fire ring, and screened porch.

Where to find water/bathrooms: A vault toilet is adjacent to the cabin area parking lot, and a seasonal restroom and showers are nearby in the adjacent campground. Seasonal water is available in the campground behind the *Loon Nest* cabin, just across from campsite 5.

Reservations/fees: 866-857-2757; www.dnr.state.mn.us; Sun.–Thurs. $60/night; Fri.–Sat. $70/night.

Restrictions: No cooking, pets, or smoking.

GPS: Entrance to cabin cul-de-sac inside park, 46.001866, -95.337791

Key information: 2601 County Road 38 NE, Carlos, MN 56319, 320-852-7200, www.dnr.state.mn.us/state_parks/lake_carlos/index.html

Area activities/attractions: The park features year-round naturalist programs, a swimming beach, fishing and paddling (with paddling gear available for rent), 17 miles of hiking trails, 9 miles of equestrian and snowmobile trails, 6 miles of classic style cross-country skiing trails, and snowshoeing opportunities.

Notes: The state park's four cabins are grouped just inside the entrance to the upper campground; you'll find them just after you enter the loop from the main park road. *Raccoon Hollow* is the first cabin in the cluster and is tucked back under the shady canopy of the hardwood trees. Wheelchair-accessible *Frog Pond* sits next to the first cabin in a bit more open surroundings. It looks directly across the driveway to neighboring *Loon Nest* cabin.

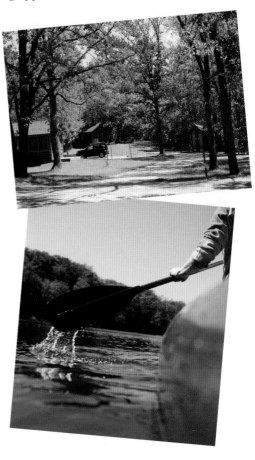

The *Eagle Aerie* cabin is found beyond the end of the parking lot at the head of the cul-de-sac. It is perched on the crest of a small hill with a view back down to the other three cabins. *Loon Nest* faces inward, while its "backyard" is a few short yards from the roadway of the first campground loop. It's the most exposed and therefore the least private of the four. Still, the four cabins enjoy open lawns with a nice array of mature hardwood shade trees nearby.

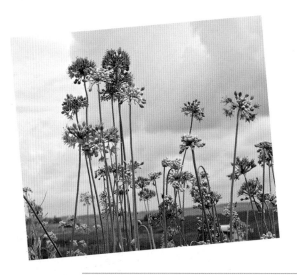

The arrangement of cabins is like a community sharing a woodsy neighborhood. Grassy front and side yards, some with a scattering of oaks and other hardwoods providing shade, complement each cabin in the cluster.

At more than 6 miles long and 1 mile wide in places, and with more than 14 miles of shoreline, Lake Carlos is the largest lake in the region. Reaching a depth of 150 feet, it is also one of the deeper lakes in Minnesota.

TOM'S TIPS: The region around Lake Carlos (and further south at Kensington) is reputed to have been visited by Vikings more than 500 years ago. The famous, and controversial, "Kensington Runestone" is alleged to be covered with (contestable) Viking inscriptions. It is now on display at the Kensington Runestone Museum in nearby Alexandria, Minnesota.

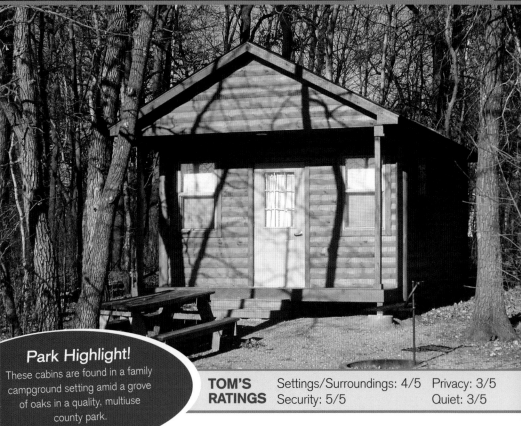

Park Highlight!

These cabins are found in a family campground setting amid a grove of oaks in a quality, multiuse county park.

TOM'S RATINGS
Settings/Surroundings: 4/5   Privacy: 3/5
Security: 5/5   Quiet: 3/5

Number of cabins/availability: 3, seasonal (May 1–Sept. 30).

Cabin sleeping capacity: 5

Cabin features: Electricity, ceiling fan, table and chairs, bunk beds (3 twin, 1 queen), fire ring, and picnic table; Cabins K and D are ADA accessible.

Where to find water/bathrooms: Water is available throughout the campground, in the ADA-accessible shower house, and at a drinking water source at the entrance to the campground behind the caretaker's house/office. The restroom is also located in the southernmost campground loop.

Reservations/fees: 320-276-8864, cash or check only/no credit cards accepted. First night deposit upon reservation; balance upon arrival; 3-day minimum rental. $45/day, with a $45 damage deposit.

Restrictions: No pets in cabins.

GPS: Entrance to park/and the south campground, 45.325984, -94.734317

Key information: Lake Koronis Regional Park and Campground, 51625 CSAH 20, Paynesville, MN 56362, 320-276-8843, www.co.meeker.mn.us/Facilities/Facility/Details/Lake-Koronis-Regional-Park-4

Area activities/attractions: Lake Koronis is perfect for a wide variety of water sports, including fishing, paddling, and boating, etc. To access the lake, head to the shoreside section of the regional park across the highway from the campground and cabins. The park itself has a picnic area and pavilion, a tent area, an observation tower, a beach, a boat landing, ball fields and volleyball courts (with gear available to check out), and short hiking trails. The area adjacent to the campground features a nature area for birding and spotting wildflowers.

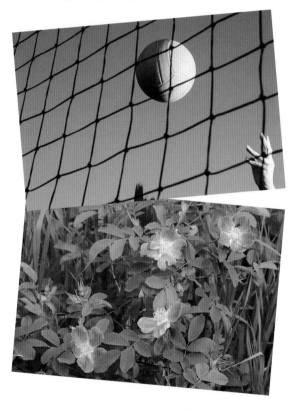

Notes: Upon first entering the campground section of this regional park, you'll encounter the caretaker's house, a few outbuildings, a gravel parking area, and a shower building, all of which is the hub of the well-maintained campground. The cabins are a bonus feature in an already pleasant regional county park setting.

The atmosphere quickly becomes more pastoral as you head towards the three cabins here. They are scattered among the campsites and RV sites in this oak-forested campground. Rustic and homey, Cabin K is within one of the five campsite loops and is ADA accessible, Cabins D and F are in a section that offers tent sites.

What makes these cabins especially appealing is that this campground is part of a larger complex that is rife with recreational opportunities. A short walk across the highway takes one from acorns crunching underfoot to open lawns and then the roadways and trails that wind along the southern shore of Lake Koronis. The observation tower in the park isn't to be missed, as it offers a bird's-eye view of the western section of the lake.

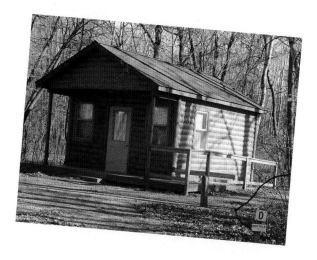

Lake Koronis is an impressive lake to behold too. It's more than 130 feet deep and a hub of boating and fishing opportunities. Canoers and kayakers might enjoy a short paddle out to 2nd Island, which is a mile from the regional park. The island features a few trails, a small dock, and a picnic area and shelter.

TOM'S TIPS: Bikers and hikers can enjoy more than 25 miles of trails in the area, including a loop around Lake Koronis and a connection with the Glacial Lakes State Trail. To reach it, you'll need to head a few miles north to Paynesville; the Glacial Lakes trail goes west to the city of Willmar.

Lake Maria State Park

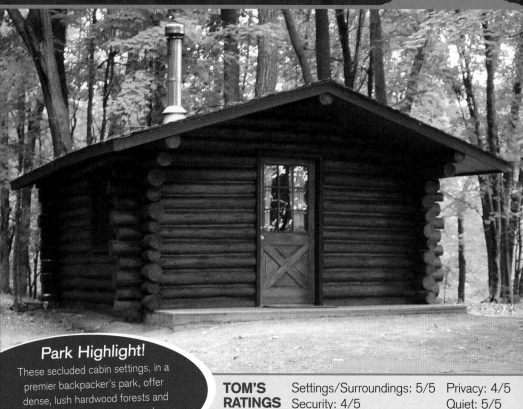

Park Highlight!
These secluded cabin settings, in a premier backpacker's park, offer dense, lush hardwood forests and challenging trails across, up, and over glacial hills and valleys.

TOM'S RATINGS   Settings/Surroundings: 5/5   Privacy: 4/5
       Security: 4/5   Quiet: 5/5

Number of cabins/availability: 3; 2 year-round, 1 seasonal.

Cabin sleeping capacity: 6

Cabin features: No electricity, woodstove heat, bunk beds, and table and benches.

Where to find water/bathrooms: Vault toilets are located at each cabin site; if you're in Cabins 1 or 2, water is available at the parking lot; the closest water to Cabin 3 is at the park office. Water is available year-round at the park office, the group camp parking area, and the Trail Center. A flush toilet is available year-round at the Trail Center; there are no shower facilities in the park.

Reservations/fees: 866-857-2757; www.dnr.state.mn.us; Sun.–Thurs. $55/night; Fri.–Sat. $65/night.

Restrictions: No cooking, pets, or smoking.

GPS: Parking area for Cabins 1 and 2, 45.321775, -93.944860; parking for Cabin 3, 45.313634, -93.938461

Key information: Lake Maria State Park, 11411 Clementa Avenue NW, Monticello, MN 55362, 763-878-2325, www.dnr.state.mn.us/state_parks/lake_maria/index.html

Area activities/attractions:

The park also has boat access to Maria Lake, canoe and kayak rental, 14 miles of hiking trails, and 6 miles of horseback trails. In the winter, it has 13 miles of ski trails (plus 3 kilometers of skate-ski trails), as well as snowshoe rentals.

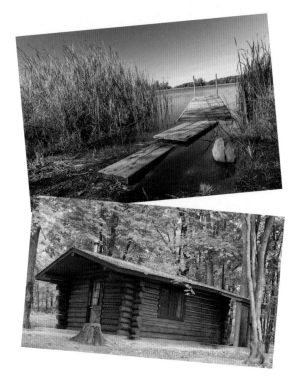

Notes: Designed as a back-packer's park, every campsite here is nestled under the thick canopy of Minnesota hardwoods that forest this park. These three camper cabins provide secluded getaways, and they are isolated from one another in pleasant, remote settings.

All three cabins are located at the end of short trail spurs that are actually part of the network of trails that wind through the park. Driving will get you to key hubs of activity in the park, but if you want to enjoy a cabin or get an insider's view of the park, you'll have to walk.

Cabins 1 and 2 are set back in the woods near small reed-lined and lily pad-edged lakes, and both are a short, scenic hike in from nearby parking areas. Cabin 3 requires the farthest walk (from the parking area at the Trail Center complex).

What Lake Itasca is to pines, Lake Maria is to the stately oaks and maples that make up the lush forests in this park. Upon seeing Cabin 2 as I came up over the rise on the trail approaching the cabin, I immediately added it to my short list of favorite cabin sites.

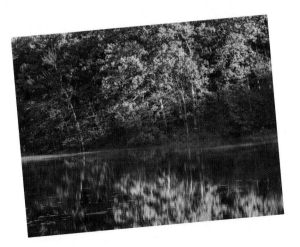

One word of caution: Visiting the park in early July, I encountered annoying deer flies in addition to mosquitoes. Expect the same in this classic primitive backcountry setting, and take appropriate precautions (bug spray is a must).

TOM'S TIPS: The trails here wind up and over hills and ridge lines, and each cabin is just a few steps from long trail loops that pass through maples, oaks, and occasional birch. Some trails are shared with horseback riders. The park's cozy cabins and its glacial terrain provide the perfect landscape and backpacking, hiking, or skiing.

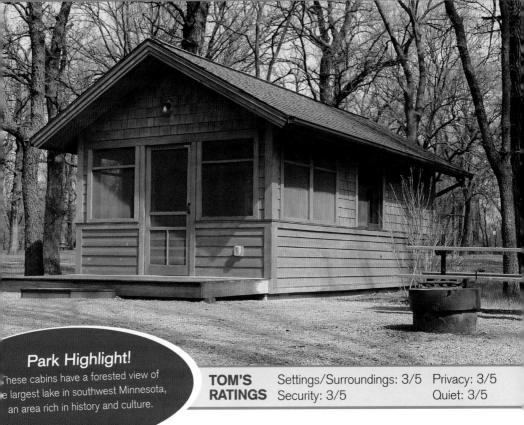

Park Highlight!
These cabins have a forested view of the largest lake in southwest Minnesota, an area rich in history and culture.

TOM'S RATINGS
Settings/Surroundings: 3/5   Privacy: 3/5
Security: 3/5   Quiet: 3/5

Number of cabins/availability: 4; year-round. Cabins are available daily Apr.–Oct., Thurs.–Sun. in winter.

Cabin sleeping capacity: Cabins C2 and C3 sleep 5 and are wheelchair accessible; Cabins C1 and C4 sleep 6.

Cabin features: Electricity, heat, table and porches, bunk beds, fire ring, picnic table, and screened porch.

Where to find water/bathrooms: There is a water faucet across the roadway from C1 and C2; a toilet is adjacent to the parking lot near C1; there is ample parking beyond C1 at the start of the cabin loop off the main park road. Showers and flush toilets are nearby in Oakwoods Campground.

Reservations/fees: 866-857-2757; www.dnr.state.mn.us; Sun.–Thurs. $60/night; Fri.–Sat. $70/night.

Restrictions: No cooking, pets, or smoking.

GPS: Entrance to cabin loop, 44.102606, -95.696118

Key information: Lake Shetek State Park, 163 State Park Road, Currie, MN 56123, 507-763-32356, www.dnr.state.mn.us/state_parks/lake_shetek/index.html

Area activities/attractions: The park office offers seasonal rentals of rowboats, canoes, single and tandem kayaks, stand-up paddleboards, and paddleboats, as well as snowshoes in the winter. It also has equipment you can borrow for free, including volleyballs, horseshoes, kid's discovery kits, birding kits, and GPS units for geocaching. The park also has a swimming beach, a fishing dock, boat access, and other amenities at the Oakwoods Campground, which is adjacent to the cabins.

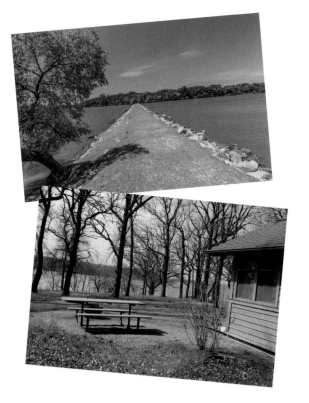

Notes: Cabins C1 and C2 are on the eastern end of a short loop beyond the Oak Woods campground, and they have a view of the lake through the trees and are close to one of the many trailheads in the park. Cabins C3 and C4 are immediately across the road from the edge of the campground. C3 also has a partial view of the lake in the distance; C4 is directly across from one of the campground loops near the intersection of the main park road and is probably the least private of the four units. There is ample parking at each cabin as well as parking areas nearby. Each site includes a spacious yard with a few scattered shade trees, giving each cabin an open, airy atmosphere.

The park features 8 miles of hiking trails and 6 miles of paved bike trails, including a trailhead for the Casey Jones State Trail that connects the park with the town of Currie, just 6 miles away. The trail goes past several of the park's historic sites from the U.S.-Dakota War of 1862, including a site where settlers were massacred.

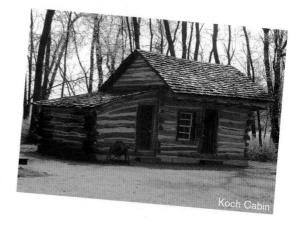

Koch Cabin

The trail also leads past beautiful views of Smith Lake and Lake Shetek, through restored prairie areas, and along several rolling landscapes of grassland and farm fields. The trail network includes 7.5 miles of wheelchair-accessible trails as well.

Winter cabin enthusiasts can enjoy 5 miles of groomed snowmobile trails. A trail shelter with a woodstove is available, and there's a warming house in the park's stone shelter.

TOM'S TIPS: To see what real cabin living might have been like, visit the Koch Cabin; it's right along the park road beyond the campground. It was the home to one of the Lake Shetek area's earliest settlers. The park is also home to other cabin sites from early settlers; they are marked with interpretive signs. Also check out The Shetek monument, a memorial to the 14 settlers who are buried there.

Maplewood State Park

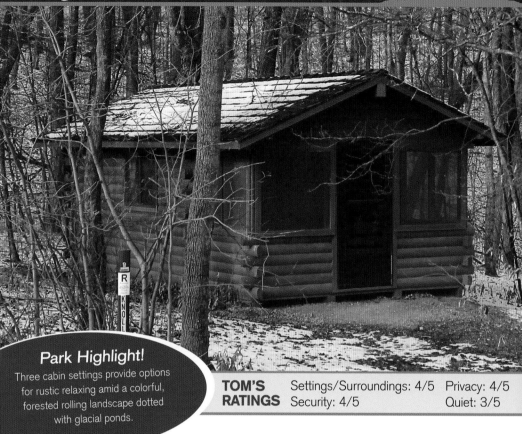

Park Highlight!

Three cabin settings provide options for rustic relaxing amid a colorful, forested rolling landscape dotted with glacial ponds.

TOM'S RATINGS Settings/Surroundings: 4/5 Privacy: 4/5
Security: 4/5 Quiet: 3/5

Number of cabins/availability: 5; 3 year-round, 2 seasonal.

Cabin sleeping capacity: Each cabin sleeps 6.

Cabin features: 3 year-round cabins and 1 seasonal cabin with electricity; plus 1 seasonal cabin without electricity, table/bench, bunk beds, fire ring, and picnic table.

Where to find water/bathrooms: Water is available seasonally at each cabin; it's also available year-round at the park office when it's open. There is a vault toilet at the parking lot of the three year-round cabins, as well as near the *Baker* cabin in the main campground. Water, showers, and restrooms are available seasonally in the main campground group. The *Knoll* cabin has seasonal water available at the nearby parking turnout, and there are vault toilets off the campground loop.

Reservations/fees: 866-857-2757; dnr.state.mn.us

Basic cabins (no electricity): Sun.–Thurs. $55/night; Fri.–Sat. $65/night

Cabins with electricity (electricity and/or heat): Sun.–Thurs. $60/night; Fri.–Sat. $70/night

Restrictions: No cooking, pets, or smoking.

GPS: Entrance to park, 46.549934, -95.954488; entrance to year-round cabin sites, 46.524057, -95.940236; cabin in Knoll campground loop, 46.523557, -95.949124; entrance to main campground/*Baker* cabin, 46.523286, -95.941061

Key information: Maplewood State Park, 39721 Park Entrance Road, Pelican Rapids, MN 56572-7723, 218-863-8383, www.dnr.state.mn.us/state_parks/maplewood/index.html

Area activities/attractions:

The park boasts a campground, equestrian camp, swimming beach, boating and paddling, a picnic area, fishing opportunities, and a scenic park drive. It has 25 miles of hiking trails and 20 miles of equestrian trails; in winter, there are 20 miles of groomed cross-country trails and 20 miles of snowmobile trails. The park is also located in the heart of west-central Minnesota's lake country, an area always popular with tourists.

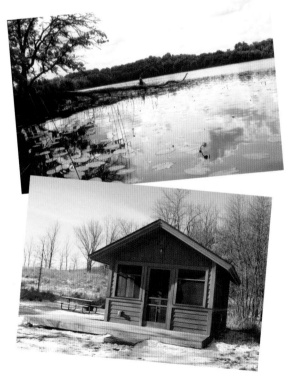

Notes: The impressive hardwood forest-covered hills at this park, coupled with its grasslands dotted with lakes and ponds, make just driving along the park road a scenic, enjoyable experience. Cabin campers visiting the park have three options among the five cabins, each of which offers a slightly more rustic experience than the next.

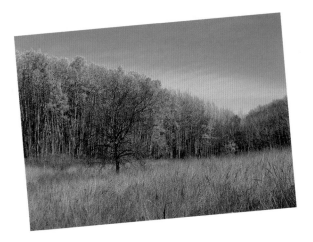

First is the *Baker* cabin. Right at the edge of the main campground loop on Grass Lake, it's in close proximity to all the campground amenities, so it's the least remote/rustic cabin option. The campground road is out the front door, and the park road just beyond a small batch of sumac out the back.

The three year-round cabins are walk-in cabins; the trails to the cabins begin at a parking lot that's well out of sight (and earshot) of the main campground. Situated along the edge of a clearing and surrounded by prairie and hardwoods, the cabins sit atop the tree and shrub-covered slope overlooking Bear Lake. A trail from the cabins leads down to the lake and a small boat dock at the shoreline.

The *Knoll* cabin is in the upper campground, near one of the highest points in the park, surrounded by a thick stand of maples that covers the slopes up to a nearby crest and also sweeps down to the shores of the lake.

All the cabins are located near access points to the park's vast trail system, which is a great way to enjoy the park's expansive stands of maples, its pristine lakes, and the tranquil rolling terrain.

TOM'S TIPS: While each cabin's setting varies, they are all located right off the park's scenic drive, which is a great place to spot deer and other wildlife near dawn and dusk. Maplewood State Park is also wildly popular in autumn; consider a cabin here when fall colors are at their peak, but make your reservations well in advance!

Mille Lacs Kathio State Park

Park Highlight!

Located in the fourth-largest park in the state, the cabins here are set back beneath towering northern Minnesota hardwoods

TOM'S RATINGS

Settings/Surroundings: 4/5 Privacy: 3/5
Security: 3/5 Quiet: 3/5

Number of cabins/availability: 5; year-round.

Cabin sleeping capacity: Cabins 1–3 and 5 sleep 6; Cabin 4 is handicapped-accessible and sleeps 5.

Cabin features: Electricity, heat, table and benches, bunk beds, and screened porch.

Where to find water/bathrooms: Water is available at the end of the cabin road just beyond cabin 5 and across the road from cabin 1; there is a vault toilet at the end of the cabin road, and it's located in the parking lot for the walk-in campsites; restrooms and showers are located in the nearby Petaga Campground.

Reservations/fees: 866-857-2757; www.dnr.state.mn.us; Sun.–Thurs. $60/night; Fri.–Sat. $70/night.

Restrictions: No cooking, pets, or smoking.

GPS: Cabin road entrance, 46.128652, -93.767906

Key information: Mille Lacs Kathio State Park, 15066 Kathio State Park Road, Onamia, MN 56359, 320-532-3523, www.dnr.state.mn.us/state_parks/mille_lacs_kathio/index.html

Area activities/attractions: The park offers 35 miles of hiking trails, a swimming beach, boat rentals for river and lake use; 22 miles of ski trails; 19 miles of snowmobile trails; and a 100-foot observation tour (summer access only). A fish-cleaning building is located at the entrance to the cabin section of the campground.

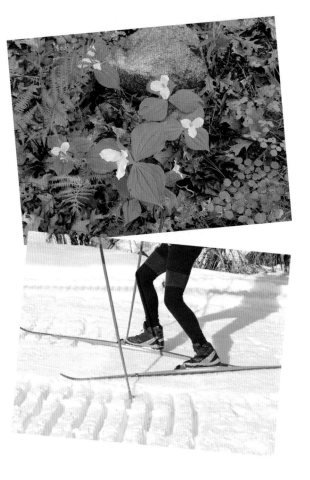

Notes: These cabins are spread out within the northern section of the Petaga Campground, which shares a wooded area with two walk-in campsites and a small hub of tent sites that radiate out from a small driveway circle behind the cabins. Cabin 5 offers the most privacy and seclusion, but all of the cabins are set back into the cover of the tall maples and other hardwoods foresting this part of the park.

My least favorite cabin site is 1 because its backyard is very close to the back of the campsite in the adjacent camping loop. In its defense, all of the other four cabins face the road (at the end of long driveways), but the front door of Cabin 1 opens up towards the hardwood understory, separating it from 2 and thus providing a bit of privacy. All the cabins have spacious, shaded yards to enjoy.

The small, abrupt hills that typify the landscape here are the result of massive glacial activity during the last ice age. The glaciers left behind evidence of their passage throughout the park, and the best way to see their impact is perhaps from atop the fire tower observation site about 3 miles from the cabin site.

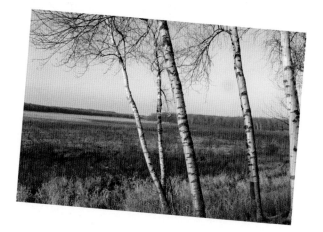

Inhabited for more than 9,000 years, this park and the surrounding area are rich in culture and history. The park's Petaga Point, now part of a picnic area, is one of the more famous archaeological sites in Minnesota and has helped archaeologists learn much about the Dakota people—many stone and copper artifacts have been found here, as well as the foundations of a house dating back about 800 years.

TOM'S TIPS: The fall colors here are remarkable, and the spring can be lovely too. For a short time in the spring, the understory becomes a carpet of beautiful trillium flowers, and pockets of these three-petaled flowers pop up everywhere, sometimes amid lush sprouts of meadow rue. It's a splendid time to reserve a cabin—the entire backyard of Cabin 5 was speckled with trilliums during my spring visit.

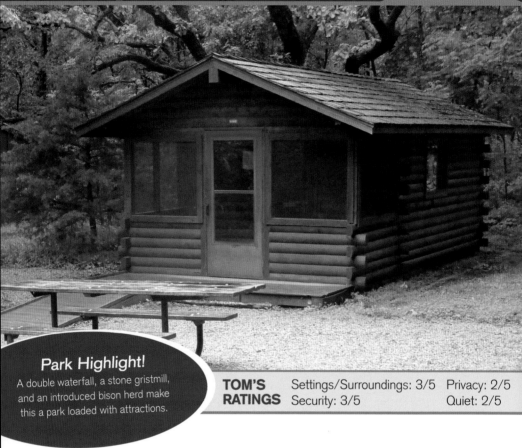

Park Highlight!

A double waterfall, a stone gristmill, and an introduced bison herd make this a park loaded with attractions.

TOM'S RATINGS

Settings/Surroundings: 3/5   Privacy: 2/5
Security: 3/5   Quiet: 2/5

Number of cabins/availability: 1; the cabin is open every day from Apr.–Oct. and Thur.–Sun. in the winter.

Cabin sleeping capacity: 5 (wheelchair accessible).

Cabin features: Electricity, heat, table and benches, bunk beds, fire ring, picnic table, and screened porch.

Where to find water/bathrooms: The campground loop's vault toilet is immediately adjacent to the cabin; water, modern restrooms, and showers are a short distance away near site A32.

Reservations/fees: 866-857-2757; www.dnr.state.mn.us; Sun.–Thurs. $60/night; Fri.–Sat. $70/night.

Restrictions: No cooking, pets, or smoking.

GPS: Park entrance/North Unit, 44.156254, -94.091432; cabin, 44.160844, -94.087592; waterfall parking lot, 44.148670, -94.092475

Key information: Minneopa State Park, 54497 Gadwall Road, Mankato, MN 56001, 507-389-5464, www.dnr.state.mn.us/state_parks/minneopa/trails.html

Area activities/attractions: The waterfall and other amenities are located in the park's lower unit, less than a mile from the entrance to the northern unit. It's located just south on County Road 117 and boasts 4.5 miles of trails and access to Mankato's 50-mile bike trail network.

Notes: Minneopa's lone cabin sits on the outside edge of the campground loop in the northern section of the park. It's a roomy site set back in the trees and offers shade and a bit of distance from the road and other campers. The vault toilet is immediately adjacent to the cabin, so expect visitors throughout your stay. Fortunately, the cabin backs onto an undeveloped wooded area.

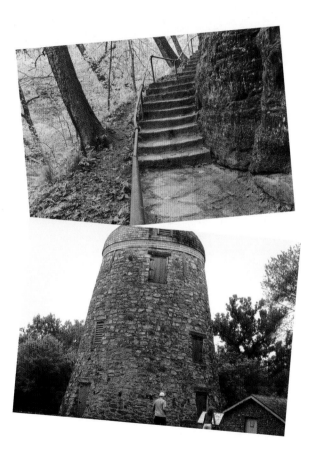

In the northern part of the park, an oak-savanna terrain dominates, making it an ideal location for the recent reintroduction of the plains bison herd that is found in a designated area just west of the campground. This herd is a genetically pure strain—it never interbred with cattle— and the reintroduction is both a sustainable preservation project and an exciting attraction for visitors.

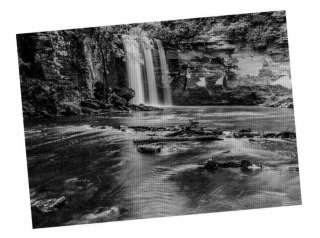

The drive-through hours for the bison enclosure are typically 9 a.m.–8 p.m., Thursday through Tuesday; the range is closed on Wednesdays. Visitors must remain inside their vehicles while inside the bison range. Hiking is allowed on trails outside of the bison enclosure. Check the park for details and other restrictions.

Other notable park features include an old German-style, wind-driven gristmill. Made of local stone and lumber, it still stands in the valley in the western end of the park. The park's signature feature is the double waterfall in the southern unit. Dropping first about 10 feet and then again for another 40, it's the centerpiece for this day-use area that also includes the park office and picnic area.

TOM'S TIPS: Severe erosion has limited trail access and viewing points for the waterfall, but you can still get down to the base for a close-up view. Be aware that the falls can vary significantly by season; of course, visiting after a recent rainfall is best. Taken together, the park's geological natural and cultural features provide cabin users with many ways to enjoy their cozy cabin stay.

Myre-Big Island State Park

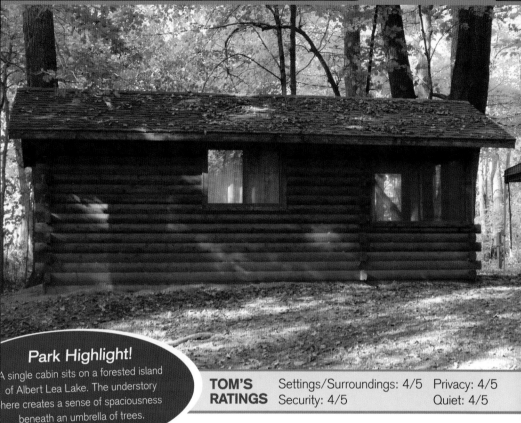

Park Highlight!
A single cabin sits on a forested island of Albert Lea Lake. The understory here creates a sense of spaciousness beneath an umbrella of trees.

TOM'S RATINGS
Settings/Surroundings: 4/5 Privacy: 4/5
Security: 4/5 Quiet: 4/5

Number of cabins/availability: 1; seasonal (generally Apr.–Oct.).

Cabin sleeping capacity: 5

Cabin features: Electricity, heat, ceiling fan, table and benches, bunk bed, screened porch, and ADA accessible.

Where to find water/bathrooms: A vault toilet and drinking water are in the adjacent campground loop; a restroom and shower are also available seasonally in the campground; a frost-free water source is available year-round adjacent to park office.

Reservations/fees: 866-857-2757; www.dnr.state.mn.us; Sun.–Thurs., $60/night; Fri.–Sat. $70/night.

Restrictions: No cooking, pets, or smoking.

GPS: State park office, 43.637318, -93.309009; entrance to Big Island campground, 43.625372, -93.293603

Key information: Myre-Big Island State Park, 19499 780th Avenue, Albert Lea, MN 56007, 507-379-3403, www.dnr.state.mn.us/state_parks/myre_big_island/index.html

Area activities/attractions: The park is home to a campground, a boat launch, and picnic areas. Popular pursuits include fishing, paddling, biking, and hiking. The park has a number of trails as well as access to Blazing Star State Trail (6 miles of paved trail between the park and City of Albert Lea). Birding and wildlife viewing are popular here too.

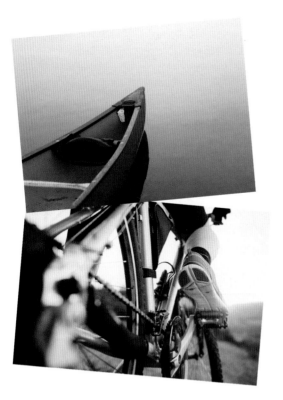

Notes: This park's only cabin is tucked into the shade provided by a dense stand of Minnesota hardwoods on a 116-acre island in the middle of a big lake. The island, known as "Big Island" is forested with maple, basswood, elm, and red oaks. This forest's location on an island has helped it withstand fire over the centuries, enabling it to flourish and making it a classic example of a Minnesota hardwoods forest.

The cabin itself is centered between the two loops of the Big Island Campground and sits beneath the shade of these lush woods. Located a short distance from the roadway in the park, it's reasonably private and found in a spacious setting.

While you don't need to paddle to reach the cabin—there's a park road to it—the park is popular with canoers and kayakers. You can launch at Little Island's boat ramp and enjoy the 2 miles of the Albert Lea Lake's upper arm, or you can cruise down around Big Island for a 5-mile paddle into the main part of the lake. There are miles of shoreline to explore.

While the cabin is tucked into the solid stand of hardwoods, other sections in the park showcase prairie, grasslands, and marshlands. Several varieties of wildflowers and other types of prairie vegetation can be found within the park. This park is noted for its variety of songbirds too.

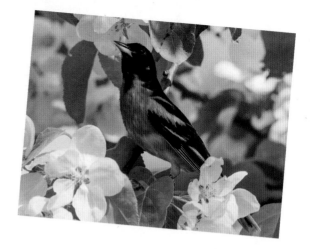

TOM'S TIPS: Hikers and bikers might find this cabin a perfect home base for exploring the glacially sculpted region along the 6-mile Blazing Star Trail; it begins in the park and then turns west to Albert Lea along a paved pathway. Other trails include one along the shoreline of Big Island, and a network of trails that runs through the main area of the park.

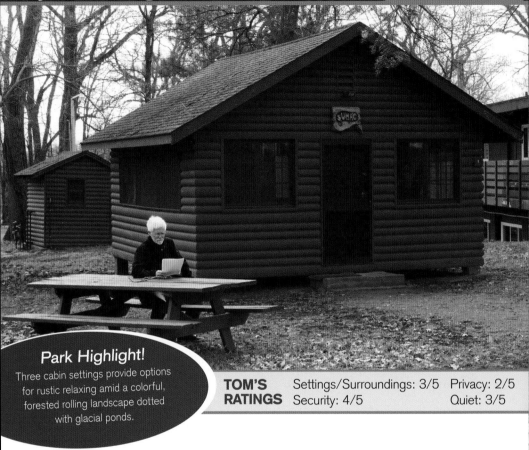

Park Highlight!
Three cabin settings provide options for rustic relaxing amid a colorful, forested rolling landscape dotted with glacial ponds.

TOM'S RATINGS
Settings/Surroundings: 3/5   Privacy: 2/5
Security: 4/5   Quiet: 3/5

Number of cabins/availability: 8 camper cabin-style cabins; 6 more cabins that have additional amenities; all cabins are seasonal (Memorial Day–mid-Oct.).

Cabin sleeping capacity: *Spruce* and *Boone Hollow* sleep 6; *Sumac* sleeps 4; *Red Oak* and *Sugar Maple* sleep 3; *Black Walnut* sleeps 2.

Cabin features: Electricity, other basic features vary by cabin; some just have bunk beds, while others include a table, chairs, and a small counter space, *Sugar Maple* and *Red Oak* each have a cot in addition to the bunk beds.

Where to find water/bathrooms: Showers and toilets are found across from the cabin cluster that includes *Sugar Maple* and *Red Oak*; showers and bathrooms are also found at other locations throughout the park.

Reservations/fees: Visit www.ci.chisago.mn.us (you'll need to search for "camper cabins") or call 651-257-4162.

50 percent down payment required, plus a $200 deposit; $40/night: *Black Walnut, Red Oak, Spruce, Sugar Maple, Sumac*; $45/night: *Basswood, Elm, Walnut*.

Restrictions: Hot plates and slow cookers allowed; no pets or smoking.

GPS: 45.346570, -92.884777

Key information: Ojiketa Regional Park, 27500 Kirby Avenue, Chisago City, MN 55013, 651-257-4162, www.ci.chisago.mn.us

Area activities/attractions: Canoe, kayak, and bike rentals are available in the park. A small historical center is located in the *Trillium* Cabin; supplies, services, and other amenities are available in nearby Chisago City.

Notes: Laid out and dressed up like an old North Country summer camp, Ojiketa Regional Park in Chisago County offers a variety of cabins. Some are situated by themselves, whereas others are clustered together. All of them are located along the wooded shores of Green Lake. The layout reminds me of a modest resort one might find on a lake in northern Minnesota.

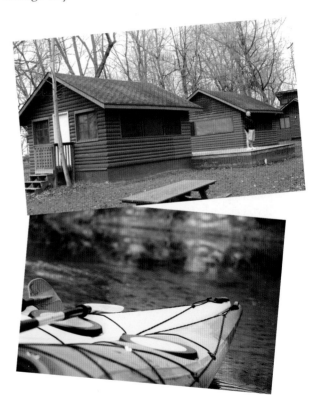

More than a dozen cabins are spread throughout the heart of this park, and more than half of them are sparsely furnished enough to qualify as true camper cabins. The cabin rental info sheet pretty much sums up what you can expect: "Cabins are a primitive stay experience. Plan as if you are camping."

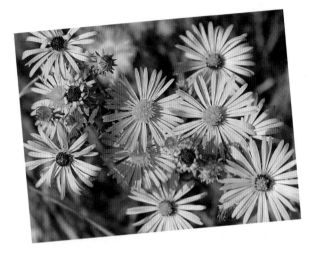

Beyond the basic bunk bed or cot sleeping arrangements, the cabins listed here offer little else beyond a table and chairs and lots of space. Two cabins share a large deck (a good choice for a big group weekend camping venture). One small cabin is off beyond the camp entrance road and provides a bit more of a secluded experience.

But you're not coming to hang out in the cabin; you're here for the park, which borders on Green Lake and offers access to 3,000 feet of shoreline. Amenities for cabin campers include a swimming beach and boat, canoe, and kayak rentals. There are also short trails that loop around through the woods in the northern half of the park.

TOM'S TIPS: This is a funky park, laid out like an old summer camp; it could serve as a movie location for a nostalgic film about a small lake resort, and you wouldn't have to do much to the interiors to get the right look, either. A large group (perhaps part of a family reunion?) might find this collection of cabins a perfect solution for a gathering. If you enjoy basic tent camping and an open campfire, these cabins are a very modest yet quaint short step up from roughing it in a tent.

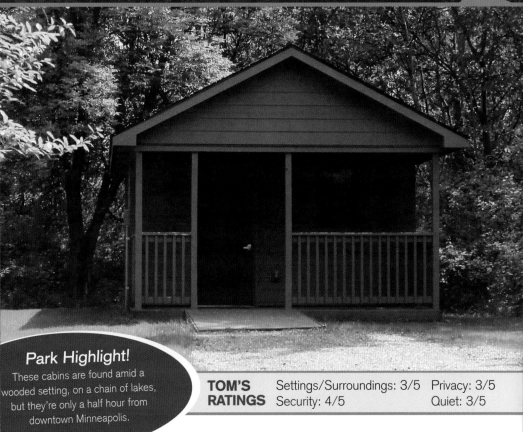

Park Highlight!
These cabins are found amid a wooded setting, on a chain of lakes, but they're only a half hour from downtown Minneapolis.

TOM'S RATINGS

Settings/Surroundings: 3/5 Privacy: 3/5
Security: 4/5   Quiet: 3/5

Number of cabins/availability: 2; seasonal (May–Sept.).

Cabin sleeping capacity: The cabin at campsite 25 sleeps 6; the cabin at campsite 26 sleeps 5 and is ADA accessible.

Cabin features: Electricity, baseboard heat, 14' x 16' units with natural pine, ceiling lights, ceiling fan, table and benches, log-framed bunks (mattresses included), lights above each bunk and a covered porch.

Where to find water/bathrooms: There is a portable toilet adjacent to Cabin 25 and drinking water is nearby in the E Loop campground; showers, restrooms, and a laundry are near the entrance to the D Loop, which is in the vicinity of campsite 22.

Reservations/fees: 763-757-3920; $55/night, $8 reservation fee. A park permit is also required; daily permits are $5; annual passes are $25 and honored at all Anoka County regional parks as well as regional parks in Washington and Carver counties.

Restrictions: No cooking, pets, or smoking; 6 people max allowed per cabin; check campground rules for other details.

GPS: Entrance to cabins in D Loop, 45.168316, -93.080900

Key information: Rice Creek Chain of Lakes Visitor Center, 7373 Main Street, Centerville, MN 55038, 651-426-7564, www.anokacounty.us/789/Rice-Creek-Chain-of-Lakes-Park-Reserve

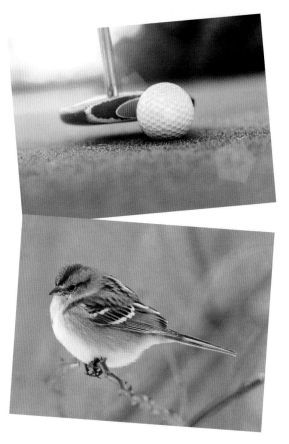

Area activities/attractions: The park features a nature center and programs, a swimming beach, a playground, a boat launch, an 18-hole golf course, and water routes through the chain of lakes.

Notes: The two cabins here are located side-by-side on a small loop in the campground complex. Each is set back at the end of a long driveway; the cabin at site 25 has a very spacious, treelined yard. Like their counterpart cabins at Bunker Hill (also an Anoka County park unit), these cabins are beautifully appointed with glowing log pine-framed bunk beds, tables, and chairs. The units are bright and literally quite "woodsy."

While not on the lake, the campground is located near the southwest shores of Centerville Lake, which is itself ideally located near the center of a chain of seven major lakes along the Rice Creek. This chain of lakes, along with a few smaller ones, features sections of undeveloped shoreline and several miles of fine paddling, starting at the dam at Peltier Lake and heading down to Baldwin Lake.

As one of Anoka County's park reserves, and the second-largest regional county park in the metro area, the 5,500 acres of the Rice Creek Chain are filled with natural and scenic amenities. The park's character is defined mostly by the lowland floodplain of the Rice Creek and the series of lakes along this section of its channel. The Chomonix Golf Course at nearby Reshanau Lake and Wargo Nature Center, located on the northeast end of George Watch Lake, provide venues for more varied pursuits.

TOM'S TIPS: There are several biking routes in the area that interconnect throughout the Rice Creek-Lino Lakes-Centerville network (though some share the road with vehicles). Beyond the park, the Lower Rice Creek can be paddled, but doing so requires skill and caution. Check water levels in advance, and watch out for downed trees, rocks, and other hazards. Birding along this route is said to be especially rewarding.

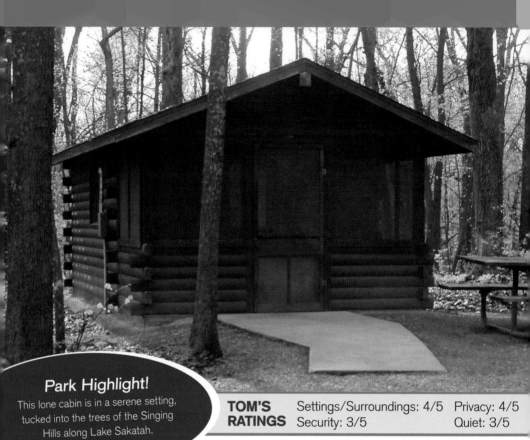

Park Highlight!
This lone cabin is in a serene setting, tucked into the trees of the Singing Hills along Lake Sakatah.

TOM'S RATINGS   Settings/Surroundings: 4/5   Privacy: 4/5
Security: 3/5   Quiet: 3/5

Number of cabins/availability: 1; seasonal (Apr.–Oct.).

Cabin sleeping capacity: 5

Cabin features: Electricity, table and chairs, bunk beds, fire ring, picnic table, screened porch, and ADA accessible.

Where to find water/bathrooms: A vault toilet is across the road; water and a restroom are available in the adjacent campground loop.

Reservations/fees: 866-857-2757; www.dnr.state.mn.us; Sun.–Thurs. $60/night; Fri.–Sat. $70/night.

Restrictions: No cooking, pets, or smoking.

GPS: Park entrance, 46.524057, -95.940236; cabin site, 44.221246, -93.537457

Key information: Sakatah Lake State Park, 50499 Sakatah Lake State Park Road, Waterville, MN 56096, 507-362-4438, www.dnr.state.mn.us/state_parks/sakatah_lake/index.html

Area activities/attractions: Camping, fishing, boating, hiking, and biking are all popular here. There is also a campground horseshoe pit just beyond the cabin, and if you're angling, there's a fish cleaning station and a trailer sanitation station past the cabin in the campground loop.

Notes: This camp is nestled under a canopy of bur oak, basswood, and other hardwoods that cover these hills that lie within the transition zone between Minnesota's southern oak barrens and the Big Woods landscapes farther north. The lakes (Upper and Lower Sakatah) are each a widening in the Cannon River.

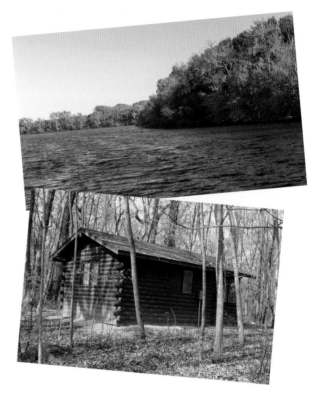

The tree-covered and gently rolling hills surrounding the lake were enjoyed by the Wahpekita tribe of the Dakota Nation. They referred to this place as *Sakatah*, which means "the sights and sounds of children playing in the hills." The loosely translated term "Singing Hills" is a common name for the site today.

Besides the amenities of the cabin's natural neighborhood, the cabin is a very short distance from access to one of the state's foremost biking/hiking trails: the Sakatah Singing Hills State Trail. The trail begins just north of Mankato and covers 39 miles in all; it's also entirely paved, making it accessible for everyone.

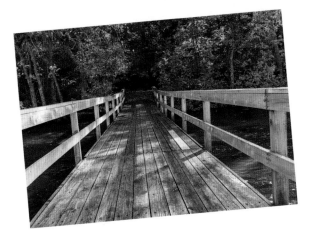

The park is also home to a number of trail loops; these include the Big Woods Loop, the Hidden Pond Trail, and the Wahpekute Trail, all of which take hikers through the dense stands of hardwoods characteristic of the park.

There's one downside about Lake Sakatah, however. If you're heading to the park in the summer, keep in mind that Sakatah Lake is very shallow and tends to develop an unpleasant algae bloom during the hot days of summer (late July, August); this makes swimming unsafe and can make spending time on the water pretty unpleasant.

TOM'S TIPS: This cabin is the perfect place to enjoy the park's lush stands of colorful hardwoods in autumn. It is tucked into the woods at the western end of the campground loop, and it's far enough back into the trees to provide a peaceful, mostly secluded experience.

"Sandy Beach" Cabin

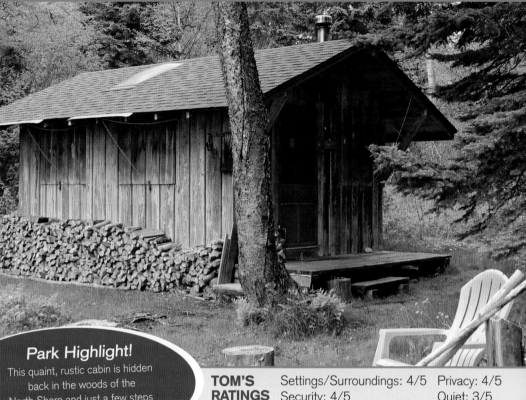

Park Highlight!
This quaint, rustic cabin is hidden back in the woods of the North Shore and just a few steps up from Lake Superior.

TOM'S RATINGS
Settings/Surroundings: 4/5   Privacy: 4/5
Security: 4/5   Quiet: 3/5

Number of cabins/availability: 1; seasonal (Apr. 1–Oct. 15).

Cabin sleeping capacity: 4

Cabin features: No electricity (2 propane lamps); woodstove for heat (firewood provided), table and chairs, one set of twin-sized bunk beds, sofa sleeper, counter space with a gas stove, fire ring, and picnic table.

Where to find water/bathrooms: The cabin has a single-seater outhouse nearby, but no water is available, so you'll need to bring your own.

Reservations/fees: Reservations online at www.cascadevacationrentals.com (you may need to search for it on the site).

Varies by season; $79-$89/day, additional guest occupancy rates may apply.

Restrictions: Pets are allowed with prior approval; there is a two-pet maximum (fee $5). Guests must remove trash from the property upon checkout, and there is no housekeeping. The property must be left in the same manner and condition as when guests arrived.

GPS: Chessie Trail, 47.820610, -90.040621; cabin site, 47.818103, -90.043180

Key information: Cascade Cabin Rentals, 218-663-7971, near Grand Marais, MN, www.cascadevacationrentals.com

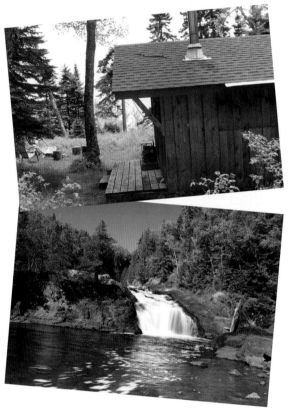

Area activities/attractions: The cabin has a private lake-shore beach and a few short hiking options, but it's also located along the famous Highway 61, so there are tons of recreational opportunities. Just for starters, Judge C.R. Magney State Park and Naniboujou Lodge are nearby, and Grand Marais is 15 miles south of the cabin. Water is available at Grand Marais Municipal Campground.

Notes: The cabin at Sandy Beach is a pretty fancy "camper cabin"; it has a propane gas stove, which is a notch up from the slow cooker/coffeemakers allowed in most "no cooking" cabins. It also has very comfortable furnishings that give it a quaint style that rises above the bare-bones interiors of most standard park cabins.

When all things are considered, this is roughing it in pretty high style. Sure, there's no electricity, no water, and a one-hole outhouse nearby. But the cabin is incredibly cozy, in part because of the smart layout: a couch that doubles as a sleeper, a modest counter area with a cupboard stocked with basic utensils, and propane for cooking and lights.

The cabin's classic woodstove is the eye-catching focal point of the cabin; it's the quintessential touch to an already cool cabin.

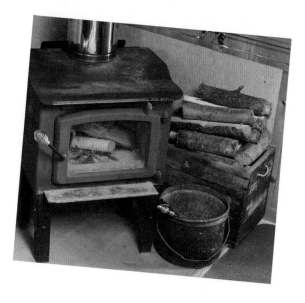

The narrow road leading to the cabin winds through the woods, past a few neighboring private cabins and up to a small parking area uphill from the cabin, which is addressed as 50 along the Chessie Trail roadway. Once you park, you've got to carry all your gear, food, *and* water down a short run of rough steps to the clearing and the cabin.

You can see the lake through the trees, but a very short walk down the sloping shoreline puts you on your own private, cobblestone-lined beach beside the waters of Lake Superior.

TOM'S TIPS: This cabin, with its private beach, sits roughly midway along the shoreline on the fourth segment of the Lake Superior State Water Trail from Grand Marais to Grand Portage. Using this cabin as a starting point for a paddling loop out-and-back in either direction makes for fantastic kayak day trips without concern for shuttling vehicles. But before you head out, make sure you've got the proper gear (including wetsuits, even in summer), check the weather, and never paddle alone. When you're done, you can return to a cozy, comfy cabin just 100 feet from the take-out at the beach landing.

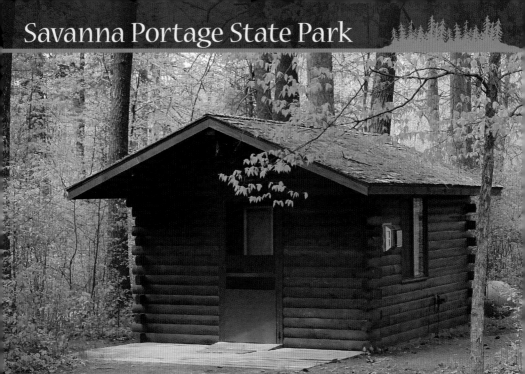

Park Highlight!

This park features towering white pines, historic portage trails used since the days of fur trading, and a cabin on the continental divide.

TOM'S RATINGS

Settings/Surroundings: 4/5   Privacy: 4/5
Security: 3/5   Quiet: 3/5

Number of cabins/availability: 1; year-round. Open daily from Apr. 1–Oct. 31 and Thur.–Sun. in winter.

Cabin sleeping capacity: 5 (ADA accessible).

Cabin features: Table and bench, bunk beds, and entry patio.

Where to find water/bathrooms: Water is just across the road next to campsite 54; restrooms and showers are available in the center of the campground loop.

Reservations/fees: 866-857-2757; www.dnr.state.mn.us; Sun.–Thurs. $55/night; Fri.–Sat. $65/night.

Restrictions: No cooking, pets, or smoking.

GPS: Park entrance, 46.818721, -93.176314; cabin, 46.827854, -93.151158

Key information: Savanna Portage State Park, 55626 Lake Place, McGregor, MN 55760, 218-426-3271, www.dnr.state.mn.us/state_parks/savanna_portage/index.html

Area activities/attractions: The park offers a swimming beach, boat, canoe and kayak rental, a dock, and boat access. Note, however, that only electric motors are allowed on the lake. In the lower loop of the campground, there's a play area, and you can access the Lake Shumway Nature Trail and Bog Boardwalk trailhead at the Lake Shumway parking lot. In all, the park has 27 miles of hiking trails, 10 miles of mountain bike trails, 32 miles of snowmobile trails, and ample snowshoeing options.

Notes: Towering white pines stand like sentinels over this lone cabin, which is back into the edge of the forest. Located at the northern end of the upper campground's loops, the location is perfect, both spacious and woodsy.

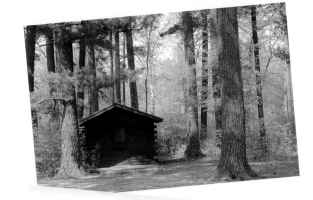

Cabin guests need only take a brief jaunt through the trees to reach Lake Shumway, the most popular spot for fishing or boating in the park. (Wolf Lake is also popular with anglers.) At the end of the lake's parking lot, hikers can head out on the Lake Shumway Nature Trail, which in turn connects with the interpretive bog boardwalk, a 1/3-mile side spur that leads off to a small lake. Stay on the boardwalk on this trail, but look for orchids and pitcher plants growing along the route).

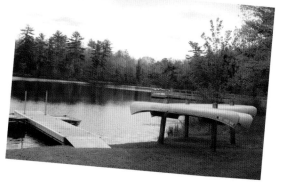

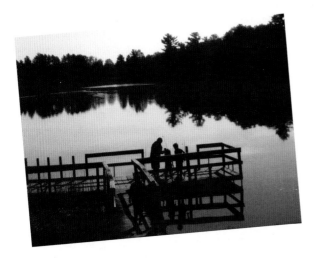

Historically, this area played a major role in Minnesota's rich voyageur and fur trading past. First known to Dakota and Ojibwe Indians, and then utilized by European traders, the park contains portions of a network of water trails that crossed lakes, rivers, and miles of bogs; this system provided a link between the St. Louis River and Lake Superior and the Mississippi River, as well as other trading centers throughout the upper Midwest interior.

Savanna Portage's network of hiking trails covers 27 miles; it also boasts 10 miles of mountain bike routes and 32 miles of snowmobile trails. Together, these trails showcase the park's natural history well, including its spruce and tamarack bogs, its beaver ponds, and, of course, the famous Savanna Portage Trail itself, which was once considered one of the most difficult portages in the entire Northwest.

TOM'S TIPS: A continental divide is the point separating two drainage basins. There are several continental divides in the country; one is known as the St. Lawrence Divide and it's located within the park. Here the West Savanna River drains to the Gulf of Mexico and the south, but the East Savanna River drains to Lake Superior and the east. The park trail that bears its name is considered one of its most scenic hikes.

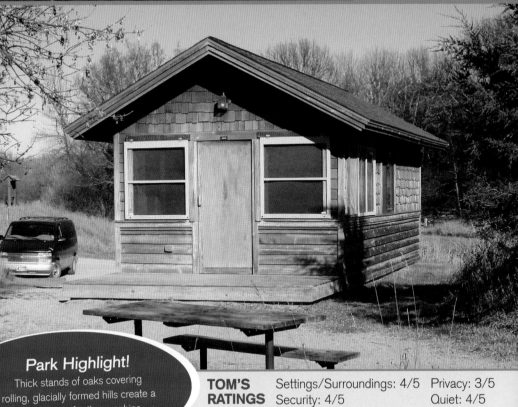

Park Highlight!
Thick stands of oaks covering rolling, glacially formed hills create a ~~li~~ ~~setting for these cabins~~

TOM'S RATINGS
Settings/Surroundings: 4/5   Privacy: 3/5
Security: 4/5   Quiet: 4/5

Number of cabins/availability: 4; year-round.

Cabin sleeping capacity: *Loon* sleeps 5 (ADA accessible); *Lady Slipper, Monarch,* and *Walleye* sleep 6.

Cabin features: Electricity, heat, table and benches, bunk beds, and screened porch.

Where to find water/bathrooms: Seasonal water and a vault toilet are available in the parking area for cabins; seasonal restrooms and showers are found at Oak Ridge Campground. A restroom and water are available year-round in the basement of the nearby Trail Center.

Reservations/fees: 866-857-2757; www.dnr.state.mn.us; Sun.–Thurs. $60/night; Fri.–Sat. $70/night.

Restrictions: No cooking, pets, or smoking.

GPS: Entrance to park, 45.311301, -95.009392; entrance to cabin area, 45.317430, -95.028578

Key information: Sibley State Park, 800 Sibley Park Road NE, New London, MN 56273, 320-354-2055, www.dnr.state.mn.us/state_parks/sibley/index.html

Area activities/attractions: An on-site naturalist hosts interpretive programs throughout the summer, and the park also has a swimming beach, boat and canoe rentals, a fishing pier, 18 miles of hiking trails and 8.7 miles of equestrian trails, as well as the Mt. Tom observation tower. In the winter, there are 8 miles of cross-country skiing trails, 6.1 miles of snowmobile trails, and 2.5 miles designated for skate-skiing.

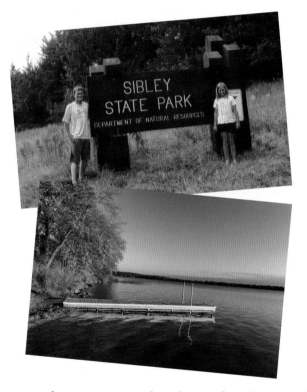

Notes: Sibley is among the best state parks in the Minnesota system thanks to its diverse landscape, wide range of recreational activities, and its well-run naturalist programs.

The cabin area here is across the park road from the upper Oak Ridge campground and situated in a clearing backed by a mix of red cedars and hardwoods. The cabins are all within view of each other but arranged to provide a little privacy.

Lady Slipper sits on a grassy knoll right inside the entrance to the cabin cluster. It's far enough away and faces enough toward the grassland landscape that it is both private and inviting.

The *Loon* cabin is ADA accessible, and its large parking lot and open space are a short distance from the *Monarch* cabin. Families wanting to share cabins should consider these particular cabins for a joint cabin experience. The *Walleye* cabin sits at the end of the cabin driveway area and offers a bit of seclusion. Happily, none of the cabins face each other, and they all have forested views from their front entryways. All are just a short walk to several trails in the park, including the always popular Mt. Tom Trail.

If you want a paddling adventure, you can also paddle a few canoe routes that require portaging—carrying your canoe between lakes. The portage between Henschien and Swan Lakes is 600 feet; and the portage between Lake Andrew and Middle Lake is 1,850 feet. If you don't have a canoe, don't worry: rental canoes are available at the park.

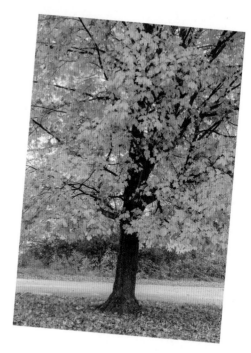

TOM'S TIPS: The observation tower on Mt. Tom sits on a hill that is 1,375 feet above sea level, making it one of the highest points within 50 miles. From this vantage point, visitors can look out, over, and beyond the rolling forested hills and lakes of Sibley State Park. Fragments of stone pipes found on this hill are strong indications that Mt. Tom offered a strategic vantage point for American Indians in the area, and it likely also served as a ceremonial site

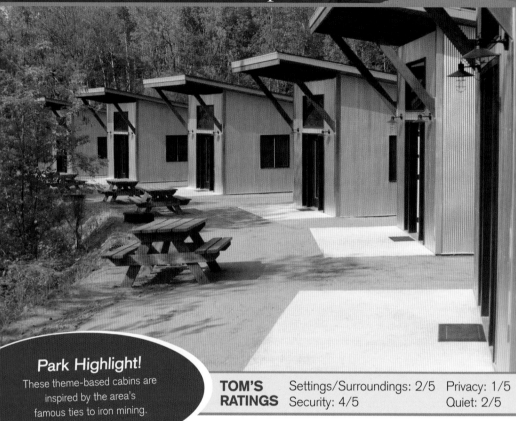

Park Highlight!
These theme-based cabins are inspired by the area's famous ties to iron mining.

TOM'S RATINGS
Settings/Surroundings: 2/5 Privacy: 1/5
Security: 4/5 Quiet: 2/5

Number of cabins/availability: 6; year-round.

Cabin sleeping capacity: 5; each cabin has 1 full bed and 3 twin beds.

Cabin features: Electricity, heat, air-conditioning, table and chairs, bunk beds, lights over each bunk, fire ring, picnic table, adjustable screen windows, high speed Wi-Fi, USB charging ports, and bike rack.

Where to find water/bathrooms: A shower house (with heated floors), high-pressure showers, a changing area, and bathrooms are nearby.

Reservations/fees: http://truenorthbasecamp.com; Sun.–Thurs, $99/night; Fri.–Sat. $125/night. Special holiday rates may also apply.

Restrictions: No cooking, pets, or smoking in cabin (slow cookers allowed); tents allowed but camping vehicles on wheels or those that weigh more than 275 lbs. are not.

GPS: Basecamp street entrance, 46.481577, -93.967296

Key information: True North Basecamp, 825 1st St. SW, Cuyuna, MN 56441, 218-833-2267, http://truenorthbasecamp.com

Area activities/attractions: The very clear mine lakes in the area provide more than 25 miles of shoreline and excellent fishing for trout, bass, crappie, sunfish, and trophy northern pike; the area is also famous for its access to world-class mountain biking trails that wind throughout 2,000 wooded acres.

Notes: Using a mining camp as an influence for a cabin design may not sound too appealing for those seeking an outdoor cabin experience, but you might be surprised! While the motif is based on this area's iron mining ties— mining occurred here from around 1908 until 1984— this approach actually makes sense, as it blends nicely with all the reclamation work done turning the area's abandoned mines into a thriving out- doors destination. Now a mountain biking and scuba diving mecca, bikers love the world-class trails, and anglers and divers enjoy incredibly deep, clear mine lakes. The remnants of mining machinery are still below the surface of these old mine lakes.

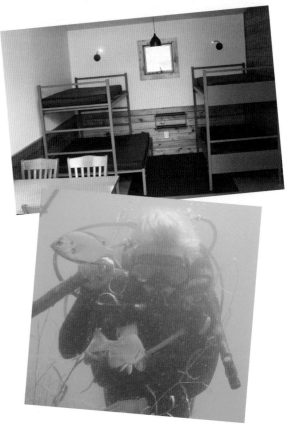

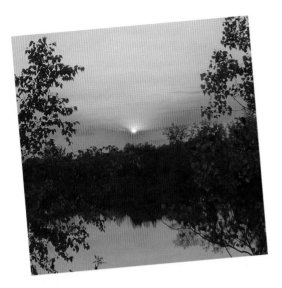

The cabins here are neat, spacious, and furnished with quality equipment. Small touches such as flex-neck lamps at the head of each bunk and drapes across the windows and doorway soften what otherwise, at least from the exterior, might at first seem a bit spare or utilitarian.

Situated among a cluster of wooded lakes within a network of numerous bike trails, the six cabin sites are spaced less than two vehicle widths apart and aligned atop the steep, loose gravel and vegetation-covered slopes that separate the cabins from Armour Mine #2 Lake below.

The fire ring and picnic tables in front of each cabin are very close to one another, making the setting for cooking, eating, and relaxing fairly small and definitely more communal than private. Happily, each cabin faces the west for great sunset views!

Because of the communal setup, this is a great place if you're a mountain biking or a scuba enthusiast traveling with a group. You can spend a weekend on the trails or in the water with friends, and then enjoy your own quiet time in your cabin.

TOM'S TIPS: In addition to the 25 miles of world-class IMBA-certified mountain biking trails, the area is home to countless backwoods dirt roads, paved trails, and just a short ride from the paved 8-mile Cuyuna Lakes Trail. This trail connects with the Mississippi River Trail, which follows roads, trails, and routes leading all the way to Minneapolis-St. Paul.

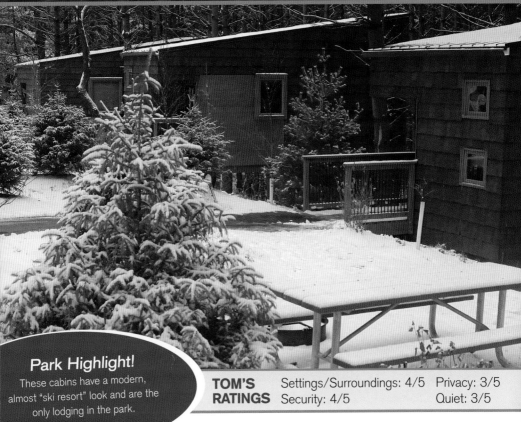

Park Highlight!
These cabins have a modern, almost "ski resort" look and are the only lodging in the park.

TOM'S RATINGS   Settings/Surroundings: 4/5   Privacy: 3/5
Security: 4/5   Quiet: 3/5

Number of cabins/availability: 3; year-round.

Cabin sleeping capacity: 6

Cabin features: Electricity, heat, ceiling fan, lighting, table and chairs, two folding chairs, two full-size bunk beds (with top rails), two multi-purpose daybeds, picnic table, deck, two Adirondack deck chairs, outdoor patio, and Cabin 3 is ADA accessible.

Where to find water/bathrooms: Modern restrooms, showers, and drinking water are adjacent to the parking lot, a short walk from the cabins.

Reservations/fees: Reservations required, see details at: www.co.daktoa.mn.us (search for camper cabins). Same-day reservations not accepted; make reservations well in advance, as these are very popular cabins. $70 (plus tax)/night.

Restrictions: No cooking, no pets in cabins; beer and wine allowed in cabins, but no hard liquor. No smoking, except in parking lot. Tents and campers not allowed in cabin area. Visit the website for a full list of rules.

GPS: Entrance to Regional Park, 44.701411, -93.087713; cabin parking lot, 44.696448, -93.088798

Key information: Western Service Center, 14955 Galaxie Avenue, Apple Valley, MN 55124-8579, 952-891-7000, www.co.dakota.mn.us/parks/parksTrails/WhitetailWoods/Pages/default.aspx

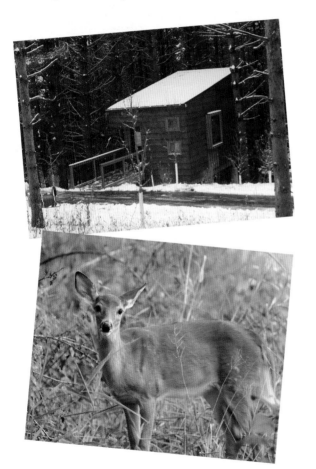

Area activities/attractions: The 456 acres of prairie wetlands, 100-year-old oak forests, and 10 miles of hiking trails are the main attractions in this rustic country park. The park also has a Fawn Crossing nature play space and connects with several natural areas that provide many other outdoor-oriented activities. The nearby riverfront city of Hastings offers a full range of retail commerce.

Notes: With a contemporary design that's straight out of a ski resort in the heart of the north country, these attractive cabins are the only lodging options in this entire 456-acre park!

Nestled into the edge of a thick stand of Norway pine and spruce, these three cabins form a modern, but quaint, cluster of cottage-like cabins and feature modest furnishings giving visitors the feeling of staying in a remote, but classy, cabin.

The cabins here are at the northern extension of a trail network that weaves through the park. Immediately south of the cabins, several loops provide short hikes that total about 1 mile. A looped series of trail segments covers more than 2 miles, leading hikers around the wetlands surrounding Empire Lake. A third network of trails weaves throughout the southeast region of the park and can be accessed from trailheads at the end of the parking lot in the central complex of the park, where

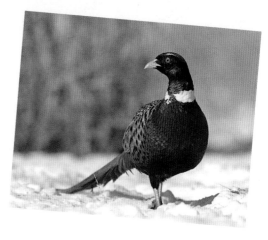

most of the structures are located. The Long Rock Trail is a 2.5-mile loop just outside the park's eastern boundary and is accessible from trailheads adjacent to the cabins and from trails off the main parking complex.

While daytime visitors share the amenities in this park, cabin users have it all to themselves at night. This solitude makes it a great place to enjoy the quiet of a rustic setting amid the comforts of a contemporary, well-appointed camper cabin, all just minutes south of several major suburban communities.

TOM'S TIPS: The plentiful hiking trails here link up with other natural areas, including the Vermillion Highlands Modified Wildlife Management Area, which lies to the east of the park and the Vermillion Wild River Wildlife and Aquatic Management Areas, which are just outside of the park's southern boundary. Both have recreational opportunities, including trout fishing, equestrian trails, wildlife viewing, and more.

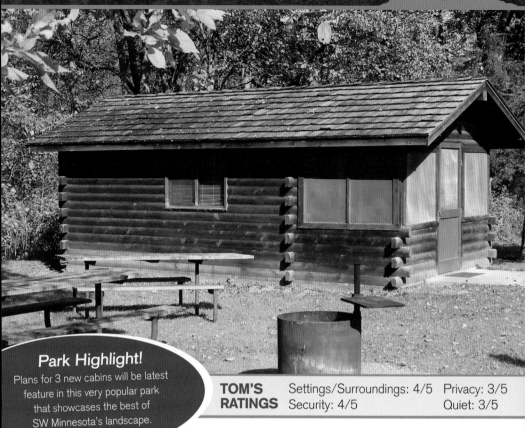

Park Highlight!

Plans for 3 new cabins will be latest feature in this very popular park that showcases the best of SW Minnesota's landscape.

TOM'S RATINGS
Settings/Surroundings: 4/5 Privacy: 3/5
Security: 4/5 Quiet: 3/5

Number of cabins/availability: 1, with 3 new cabins now under construction; seasonal (Apr.–Nov., and sometimes to Dec. to accommodate deer hunters).

Cabin sleeping capacity: 5

Cabin features: Electricity, heat, table and benches, bunk beds, fire ring, picnic table, screened porch, and ADA accessible.

Where to find water/bathrooms: Water is seasonally available behind the cabin in the campground loop and at end of parking lot near RV dump station; seasonal restroom/showers are nearby in the Upper Cedar Hill Campground. Restrooms and water are available year round in the visitor center.

Reservations/fees: Sun.–Thurs. $60/night; Fri.–Sat $70/night.

Restrictions: No pets, smoking, or cooking.

GPS: Current cabin, 44.061985, -92.045912; entrance to new cabins will be located at: 44.058404, -92.042901

Key information: Whitewater State Park, 19041 Highway 74, Altura, MN 55910; 507-932-3007; www.dnr.state.mn.us/state_parks/whitewater/

Area activities/attractions: The visitor center here is open year round, and introduces visitors to the parks many trails, the nearby Whitewater Wildlife Management Area, and the park's cross-country skiing. The park also boasts picnic grounds, a swimming beach, trout fishing, interpretive programs, spring wildflowers, and, perhaps most importantly, it claims to have a "noticeable lack of mosquitoes."

Notes: Whitewater State Park is one of the most popular parks in Minnesota. This entire region of southeast Minnesota is cut by deep valleys blanketed with maples and birch, and sparkling streams run— sometime intermittently—through these valleys creating the landscape in which this cabin (and future cabins) are located.

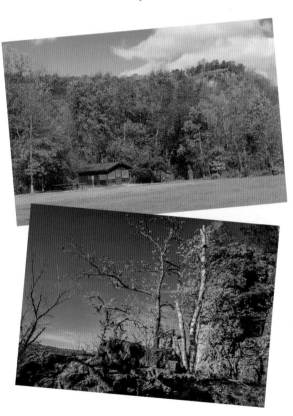

There's only one cabin in the park presently; it sits adjacent to a parking lot at the edge of a large grass-covered open space behind a cluster of trees surrounding the park offices. It's located just off the main entrance into the start of the upper loop in the Upper Cedar Hills Campground.

Tucked into the base of a tree-covered bluff that rises impressively up from the

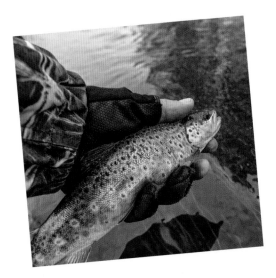

valley floor, the immediate area around the cabin is a forested setting, with a spacious side yard with a few scattered trees about. However, the view out the front door is to an expansive lawn with a circular drive path and pre-sumably the parking area for the Hiking Club Trail nearby that disappears into the forest just beyond the cabin.

Most of the park's amenities, including the trout streams (brooks, browns and rainbows are found here) and the swimming area, are within short jaunts of the cabin.

TOM'S TIPS: The big news at Whitewater State Park is the development of a new campground, including four cabins, just across the highway where the group campground is now located.

Scheduled for completion in 2017, the cabin sites will include a tent pad, nearby vault toilets, drinking water and nearby access to the picnic area, and group camping amenities (fire ring, pavilion, etc.). One site will have a tent pad adjacent to the structure and two will be ADA accessible. Built near the base of the bluff line, each cabin will have its own vista of the surrounding hardwood forest. All this will add even more to this already impressive and popular park.

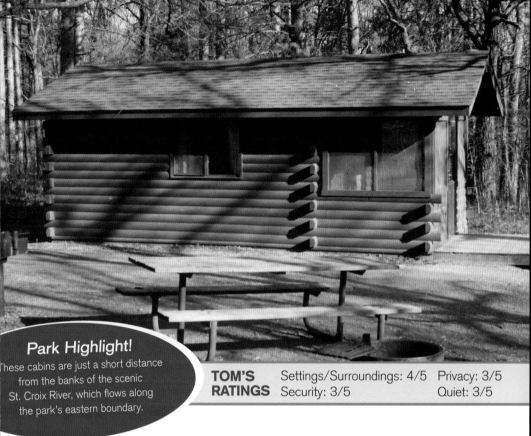

Park Highlight!

These cabins are just a short distance from the banks of the scenic St. Croix River, which flows along the park's eastern boundary.

TOM'S RATINGS

Settings/Surroundings: 4/5   Privacy: 3/5
Security: 3/5   Quiet: 3/5

Number of cabins/availability: 6; year-round.

Cabin sleeping capacity: Cabins 1, 2, 4, and 6 sleep 6; Cabin 3 and Cabin 5 sleep 5 and are ADA accessible.

Cabin features: Electricity, heat, ceiling fans, table and benches, bunk beds, fire ring, picnic table, and screened porch.

Where to find water/bathrooms: Vault toilets and drinking water are available year-round across the road from Cabins 3 and 4; seasonal restrooms and showers are available nearby in the first campground loop.

Reservations/fees: 866-857-2757; www.dnr.state.mn.us; Sun.–Thurs. $60/night; Fri.–Sat. $70/night.

Restrictions: No cooking, pets, or smoking.

GPS: 45.524118, -92.754441. Some GPS links may direct you to the geographic center of the park, Sunrise Landing area, and not to the main park entrance; road to start of cabin row, 45.542251, -92.738044

Key information: Wild River State Park, 39797 Park Trail, Center City, MN 55012, 651-583-2125, www.dnr.state.mn.us/state_parks/wild_river/index.html

Area activities/attractions: The park has a 35-mile network of hiking and skiing trails. It offers canoe rental and shuttle, the McElroy Visitor Center, and Nevers Dam scenic overlook. In winter, snowshoes and cross-country skis are rented at a concession on site.

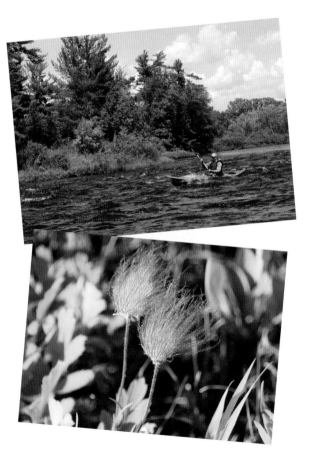

Notes: These cabins are in a line along a dead-end road and the main campground loops are just a short distance through the trees. Each cabin is set back off the road and surrounded by a dense forest of hardwoods and conifers (mostly spruce and pine). The light understory screens most of the direct view between each cabin, providing a comfortable degree of privacy. Each cabin's yard has ample room for relaxing outside as well.

The cabins are only a short distance from access to major hiking routes and a network of trail loops within the park. The Old Logging Trail cuts through the heart of a forested area and connects with several trail loops that wind throughout the southern section of this long, narrow park. More than 10 miles of trails follow along the edge of the scenic St. Croix River.

Like most other parks in Minnesota, Wild River is rich in geological and American Indian history. Ancient American Indian settlement sites developed along the river more than 6,000 years ago. More recently, commerce centers for fur traders have sprung up along its banks; roads were built to connect St. Paul with Lake Superior (remnants of that road and other logging trails still exist within the park). The Nevers Dam site was built to facilitate the thriving white pine timber industry that lasted in the region from the 1890s into the first few decades of the 1900s.

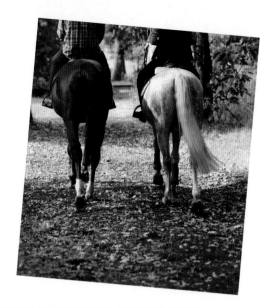

TOM'S TIPS: Bring your canoe or kayak or rent one from the park concessionaire. The St. Croix is a serene, soothing sight and an easy paddle throughout this stretch of this National Scenic River. There are even paddle-in and hike-in river camps along the way. While you're paddling, look for wildlife, and cast a line when fishing along the river. Note: If you go paddling, be wary if water levels are high or if it recently rained heavily, as this can increase the current of the river, making a paddling trip more dangerous on these usually tranquil waters.

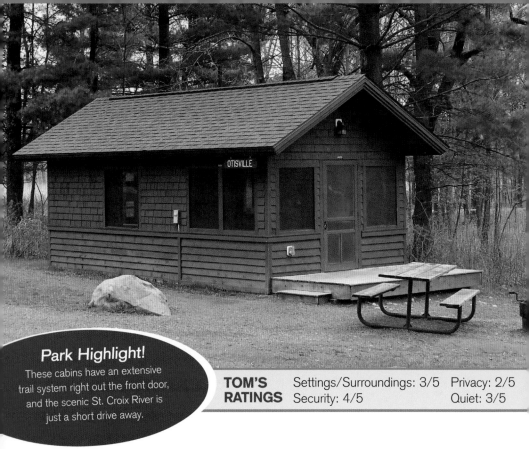

TOM'S RATINGS

Settings/Surroundings: 3/5   Privacy: 2/5
Security: 4/5   Quiet: 3/5

Number of cabins/availability: 4; *Marine Mills, Otisville*, and *Vasa* are available year-round; the *Copas* cabin is seasonal (Apr. 1–Oct. 30).

Cabin sleeping capacity: *Otisville* sleeps 6; *Marine Mills, Vasa*, and *Copas* sleep 5 (Both *Marine Mills* and *Vasa* are ADA accessible).

Cabin features: Electricity, heat (except *Copas* cabin), table and chairs, bunk beds, fire ring, picnic table, and screened porch.

Where to find water/bathrooms: The camper cabins here are arranged in a circle; a vault toilet and water are near its entrance. Water for *Copas* is adjacent to campsite 76E and toilets are nearby between the campground loops. Restrooms and showers are located between the second and third campground loops and also available at the lower campground.

Reservations/fees: 866-857-2757; www.dnr.state.mn.us; Sun.–Thurs. $60/night; Fri.–Sat. $70/night.

Restrictions: No cooking, pets, or smoking. No tents allowed on cabin sites.

GPS: Cabin loop, 45.225842, -92.772089; *Copas* cabin, 45.225879, -92.772899

Key information: William O'Brien State Park, 16821 O'Brien Trail North, Marine on St. Croix, MN 55404, 651-433-0500, www.dnr.state.mn.us/state_parks/william_obrien/index.html

Area activities/attractions:

The park rents out canoes, kayaks, and paddleboards, and it also has a swimming beach, a boat launch, and 16 miles of hiking trails. Supplies and services are nearby in Taylors Falls or Stillwater.

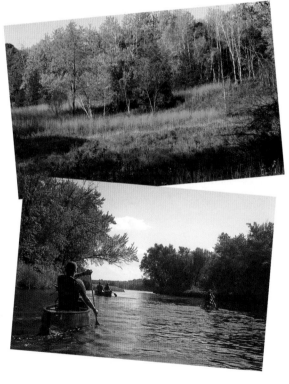

Notes: William O'Brien has two distinct personalities. There's its river face with myriad recreational options on the St. Croix River, and there's its woodlands face, with miles of trails that weave through the woods and hills beyond the upper campground.

Three of the cabins form a small circle with their own entrance just before the upper campground. Nestled into a few scattered pines, *Otisville, Marine Mills,* and *Vasa* cabins offer an open, woodsy setting, all in view of each other but separated from the campground entrance by woods and understory. The cul-de-sac arrangement includes water and vault toilets conveniently located right in the circle.

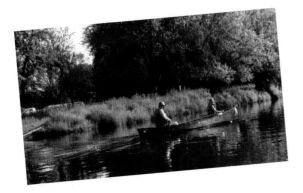

The *Copas* cabin sits just inside the intersection of the park road and the upper campground, right across the way from the first of four campsite loops, which may make it a busier, noisier site.

Just beyond the cabins is a network of trails that lace through the hills and mixed stands of hardwoods throughout the park's western regions. Expect to see brilliant fall colors in this area. These trails, and the nearby heated cabins, are especially alluring to cross-country skiers and snowshoers.

TOM'S TIPS: As a riverside park along the St. Croix, there are many opportunities to enjoy a paddling adventure here. You can either bring your own canoe (and arrange your own shuttle) or sign up with one of the canoe rental/shuttle operations serving the area. The float from Taylors Falls down to William O'Brien park is one of the most popular and relaxing paddling day trips in the state. So bring your canoe and your hiking boots and look forward to leaning your paddles against the wall and putting your feet up as you relax in one of these rustic, cozy cabins.

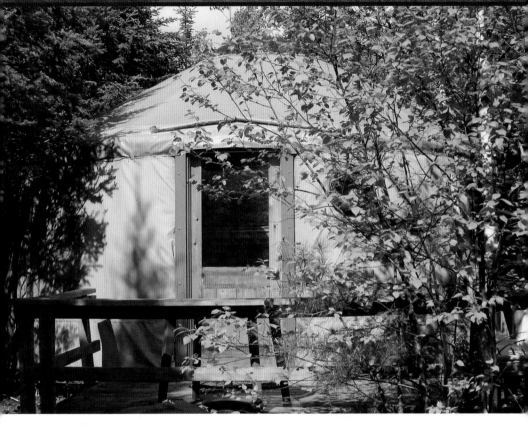

Increasing in popularity throughout the state, yurts provide an alternative to the traditional cabin. Fashioned after the huts of nomads from the steppes of Asia, the yurt is basically a framed, circular "tent" of sorts, with fabric walls and a wooden frame and floor. In our state parks, they are furnished with basic amenities similar to a camper cabin. They are in high demand, especially in winter when they are used as a home base for cross-country skiers.

And like their cabin counterparts, yurts are located in a full range of settings, from the edge of campgrounds to remote locations accessible only by foot or boat. While some yurts offer modified kitchens with a few appliances, we'll only cover yurts that offer minimal amenities here. These yurts all lack kitchens and plumbing and will only occasionally have heat or electricity.

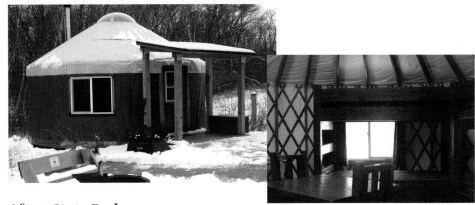

Afton State Park

Afton's two yurts are available year-round. They are located in the southeast section of the park, adjacent to the camper cabins. Each yurt is 20 feet in diameter and sleeps 7. There are twin bunk beds and a twin bed above a full-size futon. It also has a wood-burning stove (firewood provided), operable windows, a skylight, a table and chairs, a glider chair, a side table, and benches. It lacks electricity, and no cooking or open flames are allowed inside. The *Coyote* yurt is ADA accessible and has a covered outdoor cooking area.

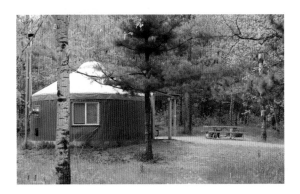

Cuyuna Country Recreation Area

The three yurts located here are 20 feet in diameter and situated on the west side of Yawkey Mine Lake, a short distance from the parking area. *Binghamite* and *Manganese* yurts have partial shade; the *Silkstone* yurt is closest to the water and restrooms. They all feature a wood-burning stove (firewood provided), operable windows, a skylight, a table and chairs, a glider chair, and a side table. They don't have electricity, and cooking and open flames are not allowed inside.

Cuyuna Country (continued)

Rates: 20-foot yurts: Weekdays, $55, Weekends, $65; 16-foot yurts: Weekdays, $50, Weekends, $60.

Reservations: 866-857-2757 or online: www.dnr.state.mn.us/state_parks/yurts.html

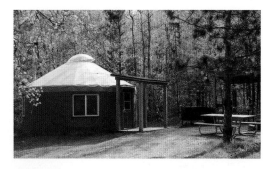

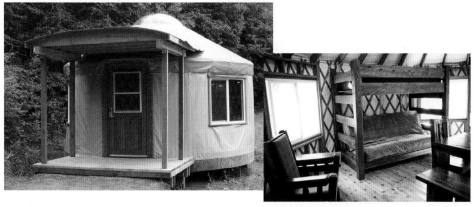

Glendalough State Park

Located on the far shore of Annie Battle Lake, these two yurts are only accessible by foot or boat. The *Eagle* yurt is 20 feet in diameter and accommodates 7. It has twin bunk beds and a twin bed over a full-size futon. The *Osprey* yurt is 16 feet in diameter and accommodates 3, with one twin bed over a full-size futon). Both are available daily, April–October and Thursday–Sunday in winter. They feature a wood-burning stove (firewood provided), operable windows, a skylight, a table and chairs, a glider chair, and a side table. They lack electricity, and no cooking or open flames are allowed inside.

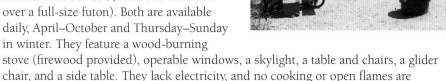

A few venues offer privately owned yurts that have limited enough amenities to qualify them for camper cabin status.

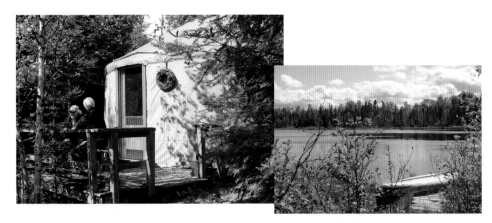

Tall Pines Yurt/Croft Yurt

Located just off the Gunflint Trail, the *Tall Pines* yurt is run by Poplar Creek Bed and Breakfast. This yurt is right at the edge of qualifying as a "camper cabin" because it has a stove unit for cooking, but there are no other kitchen appliances. Otherwise, it's furnished with the usual amenities (bunk beds, a table and chairs, gas lighting). It's in a remote setting, tucked into the thick of the surrounding hardwoods. A complimentary canoe, sauna, and nearby trails provide several recreational options.

The *Tall Pines* yurt sleeps 6 and is available year-round; it is also part of a yurt-to-yurt skiing option. You spend one night in *Tall Pines*, then ski to the *Croft* yurt, which sleeps 9 and is only available in winter).

Information/Website: www.poplarcreekbnb.com/accommodations.html.

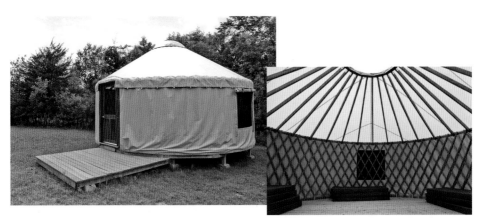

Tanadoona Yurt

This basic yurt is offered as part of the diverse lodging options at Camp Fire Minnesota in Excelsior. It offers its no-frills yurt to the public September-May. Accessible by a half-mile trail, the yurt is a basic shell offering only twin-size mattresses and cots. There is no heat, electricity, or plumbing. A fire ring and a picnic table are available for camp cooking. No pets, open flames, smoking, or cooking are allowed inside. Park facilities and amenities are nearby.

Information/Website: http://campfiremn.org

Camper Cabins Checklist

- [ ] Afton State Park
- [ ] Baker Park Reserve
- [ ] Banning State Park
- [ ] Bear Head Lake State Park
- [ ] Beaver Creek Valley State Park
- [ ] Big Bog State Recreation Area
- [ ] Brown Park South
- [ ] Bunker Hills Regional Park
- [ ] Chippewa County Park
- [ ] Crow Wing State Park
- [ ] East Bearskin Lake National Forest Campground
- [ ] Elm Creek Park Reserve
- [ ] Flandrau State Park
- [ ] Forestville State Park/Mystery Cave
- [ ] Glacial Lakes State Park
- [ ] Glendalough State Park
- [ ] Gunflint Pines Cabins
- [ ] Hayes Lake State Park
- [ ] Hok-Si-La Municipal Park
- [ ] Jay Cooke State Park
- [ ] Lac Qui Parle State Park
- [ ] Lake Bemidji State Park
- [ ] Lake Carlos State Park

- [ ] Lake Koronis County Park
- [ ] Lake Maria State Park
- [ ] Lake Shetek State Park
- [ ] Maplewood State Park
- [ ] Mille Lacs Kathio State Park
- [ ] Minneopa State Park
- [ ] Myre-Big Island State Park
- [ ] Ojiketa Regional Park
- [ ] Rice Creek Chain of Lakes Park Reserve
- [ ] Sakatah State Park
- [ ] "Sandy Beach" Cabin
- [ ] Savanna Portage State Park
- [ ] Sibley State Park
- [ ] True North Basecamp Cabins
- [ ] Whitetail Woods Regional Park
- [ ] Wild River State Park
- [ ] William O'Brien State Park
- [ ] Yurts (several)

ABOUT THE AUTHOR

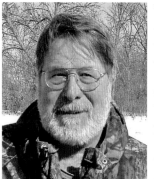

Tom Watson is an award-winning freelance writer specializing in a variety of outdoor topics: kayaking, camping, self-reliance, and more. He is the author of *Best Tent Camping-Minnesota* and *60 Hikes within 60 Miles of Minneapolis and St. Paul* as well as a book on self-reliance in the outdoors and a children's book on paddling. He is an active member of the Outdoor Writers Association of America and the Association of Great Lakes Outdoor Writers.

He is the Camping 101 editor at sportsmansguide.com and a frequent contributor for Guidelines at paddling.net. Tom's appreciation of Minnesota's state parks began as a forestry student at the University of Minnesota where he spent two field campus sessions in cabins at Lake Itasca and Cloquet. As an avid camper and naturalist, he has visited every state park in the system.